STP 1408

Isocyanates: Sampling, Analysis, and Health Effects

Jacques Lesage, Irene DeGraff, and Richard Danchik, editors

ASTM Stock Number: STP1408

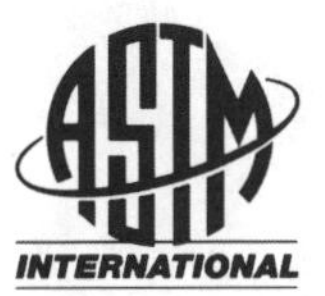

ASTM
100 Barr Harbor Drive
PO Box C700
West Conshohocken, PA 19428-2959

Printed in the U.S.A.

Library of Congress Cataloging-in-Publication Data

Isocyanates : sampling, analysis, and health effects / Jacques Lesage,
Irene DeGraff, and Richard Danchik, editors.
    p. cm. – (STP ; 1408)
    "ASTM Stock Number: STP1408."
    Contains papers presented at a symposium.
    Includes bibliographical references and index.
    ISBN 0-8031-2879-7
    1. Isocyanates—Toxicology—Congresses. 2. Isocyanates—Environmental
    aspects—Congresses. 3. Isocyanates—Analysis—Congresses. 4.
    Environmental sampling—Congresses. I. Lesage, Jacques, 1958- II.
    DeGraff, Irene, 1948- III. Danchik, Richard, 1943- IV. ASTM special
    technical publication ; 1408.
    RA1247.M45 I84 2001
    615.9'5142—dc21

                              2001056056

Photocopy Rights

Authorization to photocopy items for internal, personal, or educational classroom use, or the internal, personal, or educational classroom use of specific clients, is granted by ASTM International provided that the appropriate fee is paid to the Copyright Clearance Center, 222 Rosewood Drive, Danvers, MA 01923; Tel: 978-750-8400; online: http://www.copyright.com/.

Peer Review Policy

Each paper published in this volume was evaluated by two peer reviewers and at least one editor. The authors addressed all of the reviewers' comments to the satisfaction of both the technical editor(s) and the ASTM Committee on Publications.

To make technical information available as quickly as possible, the peer-reviewed papers in this publication were prepared "camera-ready" as submitted by the authors.

The quality of the papers in this publication reflects not only the obvious efforts of the authors and the technical editor(s), but also the work of the peer reviewers. In keeping with long-standing publication practices, ASTM International maintains the anonymity of the peer reviewers. The ASTM Committee on Publications acknowledges with appreciation their dedication and contribution of time and effort on behalf of ASTM International.

Printed in Saline, MI
2002

Foreword

This publication, *Isocyanates: Sampling, Analysis, and Health Effects,* contains papers presented at the symposium of the same name held in Orlando, Florida, on October 26–27, 2000. The symposium was sponsored by ASTM Committee D22 on Sampling and Analysis of Atmospheres, and its Subcommittee D22.04 on Workplace Atmospheres, in cooperation with IRSST (Institut de recherché en sante et en securite du travail du Quebec). The symposium co-chairs were Irene D. DeGraff, Supelco, Bellefonte, Pennsylvania, USA and Jacques Lesage, IRSST, Montreal, Quebec, Canada.

Contents

Richard H. Brown[1]

Isocyanate Measurement Methods – ISO Standardization

Reference: Brown, R.H., **"Isocyanate Measurement Methods – ISO Standardization,"** *Isocyanates: Sampling, Analysis and Health Effects, ASTM STP 1408*, J. Lesage, I. D. DeGraff, and R. S. Danchik, Eds., American Society for Testing and Materials, West Conshohocken, PA, 2002.

Abstract: Historically, a large number of alternative methods have been devised for the measurement of airborne isocyanates. Nearly all these methods rely on the derivatization of the reactive isocyanate groups to products that can be analyzed, usually by some form of chromatography. The choice of an ideal method relies partly on the requirements of the regulatory authorities, but there are also technical considerations concerning the validity and reliability of the various methods and the cost and availability of instrumentation. It would be comforting if we had a consistent body of advice from the regulatory authorities concerned. However, NIOSH (USA) recommends three methods, OSHA (USA) recommends two methods, ASTM (USA) recommends three methods, NIWL (Sweden) recommends one method and the HSE (UK) recommends two methods. All of these methods are different, with the exception of the 1-(2-methoxyphenyl)piperazine (2-MP) and the 1-(2-pyridyl)piperazine (2-PP) methods, which appear twice.

Can the International Standardization Organization help? Actually, ISO is preparing four technical specifications. First, it is preparing a method based on the 2-MP reagent (ISO/FDIS 16207). Second, it is preparing a method based on the 9-(1-methyl-anthracenyl)piperazine reagent (New Work Item). Two further methods, based on the dibutylamine method and the Iso-Chek™ method have been agreed as potential new work items but have not been balloted yet. So many alternative methods would seem inconsistent with the ISO objective of variety reduction. The reason is that, in addition to having different areas of application, all existing methods have some disadvantages. Thus, a fifth (guidance) standard is being developed which will explain in more detail the advantages and disadvantages of each method and it is hoped, will point to the development of a genuinely universal method.

Keywords: isocyanates, air quality, measurement methods, standardization

---

[1]Health and Safety Laboratory, Broad Lane, Sheffield S3 7HQ, UK.

Introduction

"WARNING - Isocyanates result in more cases of occupational asthma than any other group of chemicals. You should only use isocyanates if there are no reasonable substitutes available. If you do use them, you must take strict precautions. Occupational asthma is a very serious condition triggered by breathing in isocyanate vapor or aerosols. High exposures can occur during heating and spraying. Following this guidance closely will help you reduce the risks."

The above is a quotation from the Health and Safety Executive (HSE) Guidance Note EH16 [1] on Isocyanates, Health Hazards and Precautionary Measures. This indicates the seriousness of potential industrial exposure to isocyanates. Such exposures are generally considered to be most significant by the airborne route, since isocyanates are recognized as being potent allergenic respiratory sensitizers. Some authors [2] believe that the dermal route is also significant as contributing to respiratory sensitization, but the majority of studies on isocyanate exposure have concentrated on the measurement of airborne exposure.

The nature of the isocyanate species involved is complex, Guidance Note EH16 citing twelve industrial processes where exposure may occur, including the manufacture and use of polyurethanes and other isocyanate-derived polymers, and processes where these polymers may be subjected to thermal stress, e.g. flame bonding or soldering. Historically, interest centered initially on the monomeric diisocyanates (Table 1), as these were the building blocks of the commonly occurring polyurethanes.

Table 1 – *Monomeric Isocyanates*

Abbreviation	Chemical Name	Formula
TDI	Toluene diisocyanate	CH_3-Ph-$(NCO)_2$
MDI	Methylene bis (4-phenylisocyanate)	OCN-Ph-CH_2-Ph-NCO
HMDI	Methylene bis (4-cyclohexylisocyanate)	OCN-C_6H_{10}-CH_2-C_6H_{10}-NCO
HDI	Hexamethylene diisocyanate	OCN-$(CH_2)_6$-NCO

However, more recently, prepolymers or oligomers of the isocyanates (collectively polyisocyanates, Table 2) have been used as they exhibit much lower vapor pressures than the monomers, and hence should be associated with lower exposures.

In addition, a number of other compounds containing isocyanate functional groups have become of interest, particularly in relation to the thermal degradation of isocyanate-derived polymers (Table 3). Under certain conditions, the isocyanate polymers can depolymerize, or result in the formation of amines or mixed amine/isocyanates. Low molecular weight isocyanates, such as methyl isocyanate or isocyanic acid may also be produced.

Table 2 – *Polyisocyanates*

Abbreviation	Chemical Name	Formula
poly-HDI	HDI biuret (trimer)	$OCN-(CH_2)_6-N-[CONH-(CH_2)_6-NCO]_2$
poly-MDI	Poly-(methylene bis (4-phenylisocyanate))	$OCN-Ph-CH_2-(Ph-CH_2)_n-Ph-NCO$
TDI prepolymer	2TDI + Ethylene glycol	$CH_2-O-CO-NH-Tol-NCO$ | $CH_2-O-CO-NH-Tol-NCO$

Table 3 – *Thermal Degradation Products*

Abbreviation	Chemical Name	Formula
MDA	Methylene dianiline	$H_2N-Ph-CH_2-Ph-NH_2$
MDI/MDA aminoisocyanate	4-Isocyanatophenyl-4-aminophenylmethane	$OCN-Ph-CH_2-Ph-NH_2$
MIC	Methyl isocyanate	$CH_3 NCO$
ICA	Isocyanic acid	$HNCO$

Limit Values

Notwithstanding the wide variety of isocyanate species that may be causative agents for occupational asthma, National regulatory bodies have taken different views on setting occupational exposure levels. In the USA, the Occupational Safety and Health Administration (OSHA) has set Threshold Limit Values (TLVs) only for monomeric isocyanates (Table 4). In addition, guidance values are promulgated by the American Conference of Governmental Industrial Hygienists (ACGIH). This professional society originally recommended values forTDI and MDI (at 0.02 ppm) which were the same as the OSHA limits, but in 1986 [3], the values were changed to 0.005 ppm. By this time, HDI and methylene bis(4-cyclohexylisocyanate) had also been added. The value for methyl isocyanate, adopted in 1977, remained at 0.02 ppm and is also an OSHA regulated limit. The UK and most other countries followed the USA lead, at least initially. Thus, the UK reprinted the ACGIH list in its entirety in 1965 [4], but in 1984 [5], the HSE introduced new limits, calculated as extrapolations of the monomer limit values, but expressed as total isocyanate functional groups. This was in response to the introduction of polyisocyanates (see above) and a single limit, expressed in mg NCO/m^3 was adopted for all isocyanate species, based on then current toxicological evidence. Australia has also adopted the UK approach, and other European countries an intermediate one (Table 5).

Table 4 – USA (ACGIH) Limit Values

Compound	Limit Values	Comments
HDI	0.005 ppm TWA[1] 0.034 mg/m^3 TWA	As monomer
MDI	0.005 ppm TWA[1] 0.051 mg/m^3 TWA	As monomer
HMDI	0.005 ppm TWA 0.054 mg/m^3 TWA	As monomer
TDI	0.005 ppm TWA 0.036 mg/m^3 TWA	As monomer
MIC	0.02 ppm TWA[1] 0.047 mg/m^3 TWA	

[1]OSHA limit is 0.02 ppm

Table 5 – Non-USA Limit Values

Country	Limit Values	Comments
UK	0.02 mg/m^3 TWA 0.07 mg/m^3 STEL	as NCO groups
Australia	0.02 mg/m^3 TWA 0.07 mg/m^3 STEL	as NCO groups
Sweden	0.005 ppm TWA 0.01 ppm STEL	as ppm; Polyisocyanate not quantified
Finland	0.035 mg/m^3 STEL	as NCO groups; Isocyanate form not specified

Measurement Methodologies

Historically, a large number of alternative methods have been devised for the measurement of airborne isocyanates. Nearly all these methods rely on the derivatization of the reactive isocyanate groups to products that can be analyzed, usually by some form of chromatography. The detection systems have become increasingly complex: from ultraviolet (UV) adsorption, through to electrochemical (EC) and fluorescence (fluor) detection. The latest methods are now more likely to utilize mass spectometry (MS) or even MS/MS. Table 6 gives a summary of the more important developments, in roughly historical order, with their principles of operation, advantages and disadvantages and significant literature references.

The choice of an ideal method relies partly on the requirements of the regulatory authorities, but there are also technical considerations concerning the validity and reliability of the various methods and the cost and availability of instrumentation. These are dealt with elsewhere [*24*].

Table 6 – Isocyanate Measurement Methods

Method	Principle	Advantages	Disadvantages	References
Marcali	Acid impinger/ diazotization with nitrous acid and N-2-aminoethyl-1-naphthylamine	On-site colorimetric analysis. Similar response for polymeric isocyanates	Only aromatic isocyanates. Amine interference messy and inconvenient. Reagent potentially carcinogenic	Marcali, 1957 [*6*]
Ethanol	Impinger, forms urethane analyzable by HPLC	Separation of isocyanates (mainly monomers)	Only aromatic isocyanates (UV detection)	Bagon & Purnell, 1980 [*7*]
Nitro reagent [N-(4-nitrobenzyl)-n-propylamine]	Impinger/ glass wool tube, forms urea analyzable by HPLC	Separation of isocyanates (mainly monomers). Equal sensitivity for aliphatic and aromatic isocyanates	Less sensitive than ethanol for aromatic isocyanates Reagent unstable HPLC column degradation	Dunlap, Sandridge & Keller, 1976 [*8*]
MAMA [9-(N-methyl-aminomethyl) anthracene]	Impinger/ filter, forms urea analyzable by HPLC. Isocyanates identified by detector ratio (fluor/UV)	Can quantify polyisocyanates. Near universal UV response factor	Variable fluorescent yield per NCO	Sango & Zimerson, 1980 [*9*]
2-MP [1-(2-methoxyphenyl) piperazine]	Impinger/ filter, forms urea analyzable by HPLC. Isocyanates identified by detector ratio (EC/UV)	Can quantify polyisocyanates	Analysis is more complex. EC detector unstable	Warwick, Bagon & Purnell, 1981 (monomer) Bagon, Warwick and Brown, 1984 (total) [*10,11*]

Method	Principle	Advantages	Disadvantages	References
2-PP [1-(2-pyridyl) piperazine]	Impinger/ filter, forms urea analyzable by HPLC	Separation of isocyanates (mainly monomers). Filter option more convenient	Polyisocyanates still difficult	Hardy & Walker, 1979 Goldberg et al 1981 [12,13]
Tryptamine [2-(2-amino ethyl)indole]	Impinger, forms urea analyzable by HPLC. Isocyanates identified by detector ratio (fluor/EC)	Can quantify polyisocyanates. More constant fluorescent yield per NCO	EC detector unstable. Exposure hazard from DMSO	Wu, Gaind, et al 1987. 1990 [14,15]
MAP [9-(1-methyl anthracenyl) piperazine]	Impinger/ filter, forms urea analyzable by HPLC. Isocyanates identified by detector ratio (fluor/UV)	Can quantify polyisocyanates. Near universal UV response factor/sensitive UV detection. Compatible with Ph gradient elution	Variable fluorescent yield per NCO. Stability of derivatives uncertain. MAP not commercially available. MAP artifact peaks	Streicher, 1996 [16]
DBA [dibutylamine]	Impinger, forms urea analyzable by LC/MS. Isocyanates identified by MS	Can quantify isocyanates and amines. Faster reaction times	Non-routine, expensive analysis. Quantifying polyisocyanates requires standards	Dalene, Skarping, et al. 1996-8 [17-21]
PAC [9-anthracenyl methyl-1-piperazine carboxylate]	impinger, forms urea analyzable by HPLC. PAC derivatives can also be cleaved to single product	No chromato-graphic losses of isocyanate species. Simple chromatogram. No response factor variability between isocyanates	Impurities may give high blank of cleavage product	Streicher, 2000 [22]
Iso-Chek™	Combination of PTFE (post-reacted with 2-MP) and MAMA-doped filter	Separates vapor and aerosol. Adopted by ASTM	Short-term sampling (15 mins). Sample may not react efficiently	Lesage, 1992 [23]

National Approved Methods

One might expect a consistent body of advice from the regulatory authorities concerned. However, NIOSH (USA) recommends three methods, OSHA (USA) recommend two methods, NIWL (Sweden) recommends one method and the HSE (UK) recommends two methods (Table 7).

Table 7 – Nationally Approved Methods

Authority	Method	Reagent	Status
NIOSH[1]	5521	2-MP	Ref. HSE: unrated Monomer + polyHDI
NIOSH	5522	Tryptamine	Ref. Ontario: partial "Estimates" oligomers
NIOSH	2535	Nitro on glass wool	Full TDI, HDI monomer
NIOSH	5525	MAP	Draft method
OSHA[2]	42, 47	2-PP on filter	Established Diisocyanate monomers only
OSHA	54	2-PP on XAD-2	Established Methyl isocyanate
ASTM	D-5932-96	MAMA	Validated TDI vapor only
ASTM	D-5936-95	2-PP	Validated TDI vapor only
ASTM	D Z6451Z D Z6452Z	Iso-Chek	Validated HDI aerosol/vapor only
NIWL[3]	Arbete och Haelsa 97:6	DBA-LCMS	Ref. Skarping No status
HSE	MDHS 25/3	2-MP	Evaluated to EN 482 Monomers and polyisocyanates
HSE	MDHS 49	Marcali	Published 1985 Out of print[4]

[1]National Institute for Occupational Safety and Health (USA)
[2]Occupational Safety and Health Administration (USA)
[3]National Institute for Working Life (Sweden)
[4]Out of print, but not formally withdrawn

All of these methods are different, with the exception of the 1-(2-methoxyphenyl)piperazine (2-MP) and the 1-(2-pyridyl)piperazine (2-PP) methods, which appear twice. Some of the differences between the advice from the regulatory authorities are due to the differing requirements of the TLVs. Thus, OSHA (but not ASTM or NIOSH) has concentrated on methods for monomeric diisocyanates, while the UK has concentrated on methods that can deal with all isocyanates, irrespective of type. But there are obviously other considerations, such as the prevalence of particular industries or processes involving potential exposure to isocyanates. Also, not unnaturally, countries tend to adopt methods developed "at home".

International Standards

The International Standardization Organization (ISO) might be expected to be more objective in its selection of methods to which it appends its seal of approval. (ISO methods are recommended, but not mandatory.) Actually, ISO is preparing four standards as technical specifications (Table 8). First, it is preparing a method based on the 2-MP reagent (ISO/FDIS 16207). Second, it is preparing a method based on the 9-(1-methylanthracenyl)piperazine reagent (agreed New Work Item). Two further methods, based on the dibutylamine method and the Iso-Chek method (as used in ASTM method D-5932-96) have been agreed as potential new work items but have not been balloted yet. So many alternative methods would seem inconsistent with the ISO objective of variety reduction. The reason is that, in addition to having different areas of application, all existing methods have some disadvantages. Thus, a fifth, guidance, standard is being developed which will explain in more detail the advantages and disadvantages of each method and discuss the major causes of measurement uncertainty in such methods – during collection, derivatization, sample handling, separation, identification and quantification.

Table 8 – ISO "Approved" Methods

Method	Reagent	Status
ISO/FDIS 16207	2-MP	Ready for Final Vote, June 2000
Pre-draft	DBA	New work item proposal, Maui 1997
Pre-draft	Iso-Chek	New work item proposal, Gaithersburg 1997
ISO/WD	MAP	Agreed new work item, May1999
Pre-draft	Guide	New work item proposal, Gaithersburg 1997

Conclusions

There are a large number of alternative methods available for the measurement of airborne isocyanates. As discussed, these all have advantages and disadvantages and may be more or less appropriate, depending on the isocyanate species involved and its physical form. Local requirements of the relevant TLVs must also be taken into account.

Some guidance on the selection of procedures may be gained from an examination of those methods recommended by National Authorities or by ISO. In particular, ISO is developing a guidance standard that will explain in more detail the advantages and disadvantages of each method and, it is hoped, point to the development of a genuinely universal method.

References

[1] Health and Safety Executive, "Isocyanates: Health Hazards and Precautionary Measures," Guidance Note EH 16, HSE Books, Sudbury, Suffolk, UK, 1999.

[2] Kimber, I., "The Role of the Skin in the Development of Chemical Respiratory Hypersensitivity," *Toxicology Letters,* Vol. 86, 1996, pp.89-92.

[3] American Conference of Governmental Industrial Hygienists, "1993-1994 Threshold Limit Values for Chemical Substances and Physical Agents and Biological Exposure Indices," ACGIH, Cincinnati, 1993.

[4] Ministry of Labour, "Dust and Fumes in Factory Atmospheres," Safety, Health and Welfare, New Series No. 8, HMSO, London, UK, 1965.

[5] Health and Safety Executive, "Occupational Exposure Limits, 1984," Guidance Note EH 40, HMSO, London, UK, 1984.

[6] Marcali, K., "Microdetermination of Toluene Diisocyanates in the Atmosphere," *Analytical Chemistry,* Vol. 29, 1957, pp.552-558.

[7] Bagon, D., and Purnell, C. J., "Determination of Airborne Free Monomeric Aromatic and Aliphatic Isocyanates by HPLC," *Journal of Chromatography,* Vol. 190, 1980, pp. 175-182.

[8] Dunlap, K. L., Sandridge, R .L. and Keller, J., "Determination of Isocyanates in Working Atmospheres by High-performance Liquid Chromatography," *Analytical Chemistry,* Vol. 48, 1976, pp.497-499.

[9] Sango, C., and Zimerson, E., "A New Reagent for Determination of Isocyanates in Working Atmospheres by HPLC using UV or Fluorescence Detection," *Journal of Liquid Chromatography,* vol.3, 1980, pp.971-990.

[10] Warwick, C. J., Bagon, D. and Purnell, C. J., "Application of Electrochemical detection to the measurement of Free Monomeric Aromatic and Aliphatic Isocyanates in Air by HPLC," *The Analyst,* Vol. 106, 1981, pp.676-685.

[11] Bagon, D., Warwick, C. J., and Brown, R. H., "Evaluation of Total Isocyanate-in-air Method using 1-(2-Methoxyphenyl)piperazine and HPLC," *American Industrial Hygiene Association Journal,* Vol. 45, 1984, pp.39-43.

[12] Hardy, H. L., and Walker, R. F., "Novel Reagent for the Determination of

Atmospheric Isocyanate Monomer Concentrations," *The Analyst,* Vol. 104, 1979, pp.890-891.

[13] Goldberg, P. A., Walker, R. F., Ellwood, P. A. and Hardy, H. L., "Determination of Trace Atmospheric Isocyanate Concentrations by Reversed-phase High-performance Liquid Chromatography using 1-(2-Pyridyl)piperazine. *Journal of Chromatography,* Vol. 212, 1981, pp. 93-104.

[14] Wu, W. S., Nazar, M. A., Gaind, V. S., and Calovini, L., "Application of Tryptamine as a Derivatising Agent for Airborne Isocyanates Determination. Part 1: Model for Derivatisation of Methyl Isocyanate Characterised by Fluorescence and Amperometric Detection in HPLC. *The Analyst,* Vol. 112, 1987, pp.863-866.

[15] Wu, W. S., Stoyanoff, R. E., Szklar, R. S. and Gaind, V. S., "Application of Tryptamine as a Derivatising Agent for Airborne Isocyanates Determination. Part 3: Evaluation of Total Isocyanates Analysis by Reversed-phase High-performance Liquid Chromatography with Fluorescence and Amperometric Detection in HPLC. *The Analyst,* Vol. 115, 1990, pp.801-807.

[16] Streicher, R. P., Arnold, J. E., Ernst, M. K., and Cooper, C. V., "Development of a Novel Derivatising Reagent for the Sampling and Analysis of Total Isocyanate Groups in Air and Comparison of its Performance with that of Several Established reagents," *American Industrial Hygiene Association Journal,* Vol. 57, 1996, pp.905-913.

[17] Spanne, M., Tinnerberg, H., Dalene, M. and Skarping, G., "Determination of Complex Mixtures of Airborne Isocyanates and Amines. Part 1: Liquid Chromatography with Ultraviolet Detection of Monomeric and Polymeric Isocyanates as their Dibutylamine Derivatives," *The Analyst*, Vol. 121, 1996, pp 1095-1099.

[18] Tinnerberg, H., Spanne, M., Dalene, M. and Skarping, G., "Determination of Complex Mixtures of Airborne Isocyanates and Amines. Part 2: Toluene Diisocyanate and Aminoisocyanate and Toluenediamine after Thermal degradation of a Toluene Diisocyanate-Polyurethane," *The Analyst*, Vol. 121, 1996, pp 1101-1106.

[19] Tinnerberg, H., Spanne, M., Dalene, M. and Skarping, G., "Determination of Complex Mixtures of Airborne Isocyanates and Amines. Part 3: Methylenediphenyl Diisocyanate and Methylenediphenylamino Isocyanate and Methylenediphenyldiamine and Structural Analogues after Thermal Degradation of Polyurethane," *The Analyst*, Vol. 122, 1997, pp 275-278.

[20] Karlsson, D., Spanne, M., Dalene, M. and Skarping, G., "Determination of

Complex Mixtures of Airborne Isocyanates and Amines. Part 4: Determination of Aliphatic Isocyanates as Dibutylamine Derivatives using Liquid Chromatography and Mass Spectrometry," *The Analyst*, Vol. 123, 1998, pp 117-123.

[21] Karlsson, D., Dalene, M. and Skarping, G., "Determination of Complex Mixtures of Airborne Isocyanates and Amines. Part 4: Determination of Low Molecular Weight Aliphatic Isocyanates as Dibutylamine Derivatives," *The Analyst*, Vol. 123, 1998, pp 1507-1512.

[22] Streicher, R. P., Ernst, M. K., Williamson, G. Y., Roh, Y. M., and Arnold, J. E., , "Several Strategies for the Analysis of Airborne Isocyanate Compounds in Workplace Environments," Isocyanate 2000: First International Symposium on Isocyanates in Occupational Environments, Stockholm, June 2000, pp. 73-75.

[23] Lesage, J., Goyer, N., Desjardins, F., Vincent, J.-Y., and Perrault, G., "Workers' Exposure to isocyanates," *American Industrial Hygiene Association Journal*, Vol. 53, 1992, pp.146-153.

[24] Streicher, R. P., Reh, C. M., Key-Schwartz, R. J., Schlecht, P. C., Cassinelli, M. E. and O'Connor, P. F., "Considerations in Isocyanate Method Development and Method Selection," ASTM Symposium on Isocyanates: Sampling, Analysis and Health Effects, Florida, October 2000.

Anders Östin,[1] Margit Sundgren,[1] Jenny Ekman,[2] Roger Lindahl,[1] and Jan-Olof Levin[3]

Analysis of Isocyanates with LC-MS/MS

Reference: Östin, A., Sundgren, M., Ekman, J., Lindahl, R., and Levin, J.-O., **"Analysis of Isocyanates with LC-MS/MS,"** *Isocyanates: Sampling, Analysis, and Health Effects, ASTM STP 1408*, J. Lesage, I. D. DeGraff, and R. S. Danchik, Eds., American Society for Testing and Materials, West Conshohocken, PA, 2002.

Abstract: Air sampling of isocyanates with 2-MP coated filters is a well-established method where the isocyanate derivative is analyzed by HPLC with combined UV/electrochemical detection. We have investigated the possibility to use HPLC with tandem mass spectrometry (LC-MS/MS) for detection and quantification with enhanced selectivity and sensitivity. Qualitative analysis of 2-MP derivatized diisocyanates was performed with full scan and the spectra contained a protonated molecule with a dominant fragment containing the 2-MP derivative. The same fragmentation was obtained in the daughter ion spectra from the molecular ion and was selected as target for selected reaction monitoring (SRM). Linear detection with SRM was obtained between 5 pg and 5 ng injected amount. Corresponding LC-UV analysis is in our laboratory performed in a range of 300 pg - 30 ng injected amount. The signal to noise ratio in LC-MS/MS from 50 pg is ranging from 10 - 200 depending on which of the diisocyanates that is analysed. Ten times that amount (500 pg) analyzed by LC-UV gives a signal to noise ratio that ranges from 14 to 40, depending on the compound. We analyzed samples collected at workplaces containing TDI, MDI and HDI with LC-MS/MS, using electrospray ionization with multiple reaction monitoring. Those results were compared with the results from HPLC-UV. The MS/MS analysis gives better selectivity with regard to interfering substances. The method was further developed to include a wide range of mono and diisocyanates with possibility to screen for oligomers.

Keywords: diisocyanates, measurement, sampling, analysis, LC-MS

---

[1]Research Engineer, Programme for Chemical Exposure Assessment, National Institute for Working Life, P.O. Box 7654, S-907 13 Umeå, Sweden.
[2]PhD Student, Programme for Chemical Exposure Assessment, National Institute for Working Life, P.O. Box 7654, S-907 13 Umeå, Sweden.
[3]Professor and Head of Programme, Programme for Chemical Exposure Assessment, National Institute for Working Life, P.O. Box 7654, S-907 13 Umeå, Sweden.

Introduction

Polyurethane polymers have a wide range of applications such as coatings, rigid foams and elastomers. They are made from the reaction of diisocyanates and polyols. A wide range of diisocyanates and polyols is available to achieve the desired polyurethane product. However, the diisocyanates and diisocyanate oligomers are also severe occupational hazards which require their monitoring [1]. Diisocyanates are highly reactive compounds, and a number of amine reagents have been used for derivatization. Substituted ureas are formed with amines, which are conveniently determined by HPLC and UV or fluorescence detection, or a combination of UV and electrochemical detection. The most common reagents employed are 1-(2-methoxyphenyl)-piperazine (2-MP), 1-(2-pyridyl)-piperazine (2-PP), tryptamine (TRYP) and 9-(N-methylaminomethyl)-anthracene (MAMA). Reagents introduced more recently are 1-(9-anthracenylmetyl)piperazine (MAP) and di-n-butylamine (DBA). Method selection for isocyanate determination has been discussed in detail by Streicher et al [2].

Traditionally, methods employing bubbler collection have been used for the sampling of reactive compounds. Bubblers or impingers are not convenient in field investigations, especially not for personal monitoring of worker exposure, where breathing-zone sampling is required. The introduction of reagent-coated sorbents for the sampling of reactive compounds has much simplified the measuring of these compounds [3, 4]. The technique of this methodology is to coat a suitable reagent onto a solid sorbent. During sampling a stable derivative is formed in situ on the adsorbent. The derivative is solvent desorbed and determined by a sensitive analytical technique like GC or HPLC. This is an example of chemosorption, and for this technique to be successful, the following criteria have to be met:

- the chemosorbent should be chemically stable
- the reaction should be rapid and quantitative
- the derivative should be chemically stable
- desorption of the derivative should be quantitative

Some of the reagents above have been successfully used in combination with sorbents or filters [2]. Recently a comparison between some of the most used methods was carried out in the field for the sampling of 1,6-hexamethylene diisocyanate monomer and oligomers [5].

Chromatographic methods combined with UV detection are lacking in specificity and sensitivity when it comes to detecting low levels of isocyanates in complex chemical environments. We have sampled isocyanates with the 2-MP-coated filters according to the United Kingdom Health and Safety Commission MDHS 25/3 method [6]. In this method the derivative is analyzed with HPLC with combined UV/electrochemical detection. We analyzed the collected samples with HPLC combined with UV detection and mass spectrometric detection. The results were compared and the mass spectrometric methodology was further developed. The mass spectrometric detection will enhance selectivity and increase the sensitivity.

Experimental

Chemicals

All chemicals were delivered from Sigma-Aldrich Sweden AB (Stockholm, Sweden) if not otherwise stated. The trimethylhexamethylene diisocyanate and naphthalene 1,5-diisocyanate were from ICN pharmaceuticals (Costa Mesa, CA, USA); Isophorone diisocyanate, phenylisocyanate, isopropyl isocyanate were purchased from Fluka AG. Toluene was dried with magnesium sulphate.

Synthesis of 2-MP Derivatives

The diisocyanates were derivatised with 2-MP according to the procedure described in MDHS 25/3 [6] . 2-MP derivatives were synthesized from methyl isocyanate (MIC), isopropyl isocyanate (iPIC), hexamethylene diisocyanate (HDI), 2,4-toluene diisocyanate (2,4-TDI), 2,6-toluene diisocyanate (2,6-TDI), naphthalene 1,5-diisocyanate (1,5-NDI), phenyl isocyanate (PhI), isophorone diisocyanate (IPDI), diphenylmetane diisocyanate (MDI), 4,4-dicyclohexylmethane diisocyanate (H_{12}MDI) and trimethylhexamethylene diisocyanate ($(CH_3)_3$-HDI). The identity and purity was checked with LC-MS and NMR (data not shown).

Collection of Filter Samples

Sampling filters were prepared according to MDHS 25/3 [6]. Workplace air was drawn at 2 L/min through a glass fiber filter (Ø25mm, SKC Inc., PA, USA) coated with 2-MP. Immediately after sampling, the filter is taken out from the holder (Millipore, Milford, MA, USA) and submerged in 2-MP solution. In the laboratory excess of 2-MP is reacted with 100 µl of acetic anhydride and the sample is evaporated to dryness with nitrogen and dissolved in 2 ml acetonitrile prior to analysis.

Samples were collected in industry using products containing HDI, TDI and MDI. These isocyanate-containing products were used for gluing, moulding or painting. For the comparison study, samples were divided in two and analysed with both LC-UV and LC-MS/MS as described below.

Mass Spectrometric Analysis of 2-MP Derivatised Isocyanates

HPLC-The liquid chromatograph consisted of two Perkin Elmer series 200 micro pumps and a Perkin Elmer 200 autosampler fitted with a 10 µl loop (Perkin-Elmer, Norwalk, CT, USA).

Chromatographic System I-This system was used in the experiment comparing HPLC-UV and HPLC-MS. 3 µl sample was injected onto a BrownLee 100x2.1 mm 5µm, ODS column, (Perkin-Elmer, Norwalk, CT, USA). The mobile phase consisted of 65/35 acetonitrile/ water (with 2mM Ammonium Acetate in both) and the column was eluted at 200 µl/min.

Chromatographic System II-In order to allow more isocyanates to be analyzed in the LC-MS/MS system was the column changed to Grom-sil 80 ODS-7, particle size 4 µm 200x3mm column (Grom Analytik+HPLC GmbH, Herrenberg Germany). On to this column, 5 µl sample were injected and eluted with 400 µl/min., starting with a 4 min. isocratic mode (60:40 acetonitrile/water followed by a 10 min gradient to 95 % acetonitrile.

Mass Spectrometry-The column outlet was coupled to a triple quadrupole (API 2000 PE Biosystem, Foster City, CA, USA) equipped with ElectroSpray Ionisation (ESI). The capillary was set to 5.5kV. Added drying gas was set to 320°C. All sample and instrument data were collected by the API 2000 computer system MassChrome v 1.1. (PE Sciex, Foster City, CA, USA). Full scan analysis was performed with the mass spectrometer optimized against a PPG-standard (PE Biosystem, Foster City, CA, USA). Full scans were obtained in a range of m/z 30-1800 with a dwell time of 0.8 msec. Daughter ion spectra were obtained with first quadrupole locked on the [M+H]$^+$-ion and analyzed in Q3 in a range of m/z 30- ([M+H]$^+$+50 amu) after collision with nitrogen gas. Single Ion Monitoring (SIM) was performed for quantification on the protonated molecule [M+H]$^+$. The fragment containing the protonated 2-MP derivative [2MP+H]$^+$ was used in screening for unknown isocyanates. Individual values for orifice and ion energy were obtained and data collected with a dwell time of 200 msec. Selected Reaction Monitoring (SRM) was performed on the transition [M+H]$^+$ to [2MP+H]$^+$. Individual values for orifice and collision energy were obtained and data collected with a dwell time of 200 msec.

For the determination of method reproducibility and precision, six individual standard curves were prepared with 2MP-MDI at 10 pg/µl, 50 pg/µl, 100 pg/µl, 300 pg/µl, 500 pg/µl, 800 pg/µl and 1000 pg/µl all containing 100 pg/µl 2-MP-IPDI as internal standard. To collected samples containing MDI 2 ng of 2-MP-IPDI was added as internal standard.

HPLC-UV Analysis of 2-MP Derivatized Isocyanates

Isocyanate analysis with LC-UV was performed on a HPLC system that consisted of a Waters 6000A pump combined with a Waters WISP autosampler and a Shimadzu SPD-6A UV-detector set at 242 nm. The HPLC and the autosampler were controlled and UV-data was collected with Waters Millenium[32] data system (Milford, MA, USA). The HPLC system was equipped with a 150x4.6 mm column packed with ODS 5µm Altima packing material (Alltech, Deerfield, IL, USA). The column was eluted in isocratic mode with 66/33 Acetonitrile/60 mM sodium acetate pH 6.00 at a flow of 1 ml/min and the analyte was injected with 10 µl injections.

Results and Discussion

Mass Spectrometry of Isocyanates Derivatized with 2-MP

Identification-The positive ion electrospray spectra of the analysed 2-MP derivatised diisocyanates in this study all showed a strong [M+H]$^+$ together with enhanced formation of [2MP+H]$^+$fragment, which is observed at m/z 193 as shown in Fig 1. There are also some minor fragments that all are due to fragmentation from hydrazine-isocyanate bond as outlined in Fig 1 that might be observed. The addition of ammonium acetate will not affect the sensitivity to any greater extent but will direct the pseudomolecular ion formation from a mixture of [M+H]$^+$ and [M+Na]$^+$ to a strong prevaling [M+H]$^+$, the sodiated adduct orginating from trace amount of sodium cations in vials solvent etc. The daughter ion spectrum of 2-MP derivatized isocyanates confirms the full scan spectra with the m/z 193 ([2MP+H]$^+$-ion) as base peak with a minor contribution of the additional fragments mentioned above.

White et al [7] analysed isocyanates with particle beam liquid chromatography/mass spectrometry. With this method the molecular ion from 2-MP derivatised monoisocyanates could be identified while 2-MP derivatised diisocyanates decomposed into fragments that proved the peak to be isocyanate derived.

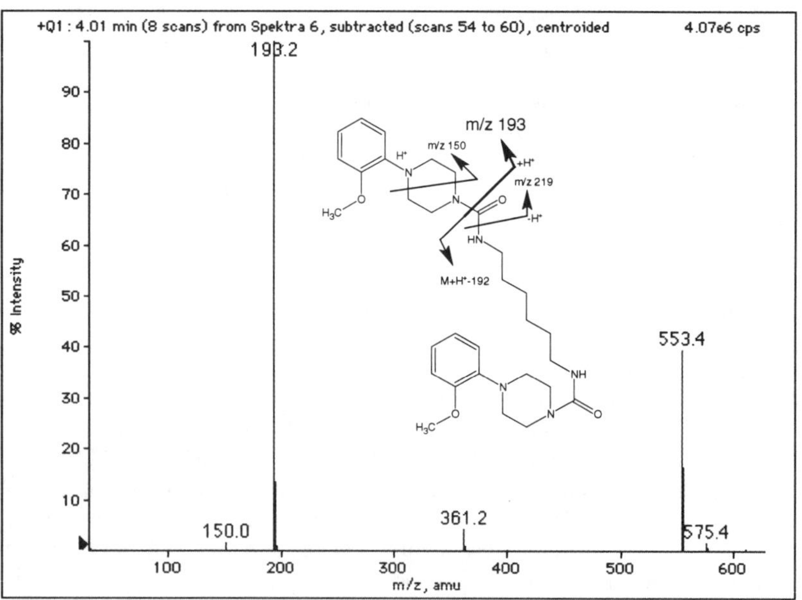

Figure 1- *Electrospray spectrum and proposed fragmentation of 2-MP isocyanate derivatives (exemplified with HDI)*

Quantitative Analysis-For quantification purposes with SIM the [M+H]$^+$-ion is selected with the [2MP+H]$^+$ ion as verification. The [2MP+H]$^+$ may also be used as a screening tool for unknown isocyanates, oligomers, etc. Further research is ongoing in our laboratory in order to evaluate the relation between the signal intensity from a monomeric diisocyanate and oligomeric diisocyanate in mass spectrometry. However if MS/MS capacity is available quantification with SRM instead of SIM will enhance the selectivity and increase the signal to noise ratio with approximately ten times. All investigated isocyanates had the transitions $[M+H]^+$ to the $[2MP+H]^+$-ion which was selected for SRM analysis.

Comparison of MS and UV Detection

Divided samples, collected at various workplaces, were analyzed by HPLC-UV and LC-MS/MS (chromatographic system I), respectively. One example from the UV/MS parallel measurements is shown in Fig 2. The figure demonstrates the superior selectivity with LC-MS/MS. The results from the UV analysis were often higher because of overlapping peaks. This problem can be partly solved with improved separation and with UV detection combined with electrochemical detection [6]. However, the superior selectivity with LC-MS/MS lead us to further investigate isocyanate determination using the 2-MP filter method in combination with mass spectrometric detection. We extended the work to involve several monomeric diisocyanates as well as monoisocyanates.

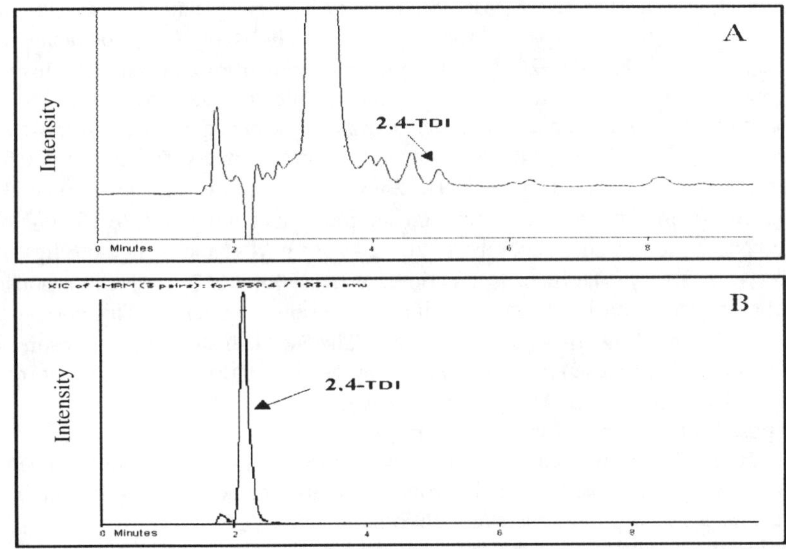

Figure 2 – *Comparison between quantification of an actual workplace sample containing 20μg/m³ 2,4-TDI analyzed with **A**: HPLC-UV and **B**: LC-MS/MS.*

Quantification of 2-MP Derivatized Isocyanates with SRM

One important issue is that the deactivated reagent, which is present in aprox. 10 000-fold excess, has to be separated from the isocyanate of interest in order to avoid strong suppression effects. In the collected workplace samples were no UV-peaks indicated in the same magnitude as the deactivated 2-MP reagent. This observation, together with stable performances of various tested internal standards are suppression effects not thought to be a problem in the quantifications as long coelution with the deactivated 2-MP reagent are avoided. The deactivated 2-MP reagent eluted on our ODS-column between MIC and iPIC. In order to separate MIC and iPIC from 2-MP reagent the chromatographic system was changed to system II. The coated filter sampling procedure was developed for diisocyanates and their polymeric products with low vapor pressures. This sampling procedure is not suitable for low molecular monoisocyanates such as MIC or iPIC. These compounds will give breakthrough if coated filters are used, and reagent coated sorbents like XAD should be used instead [3].

Due to the superior selectivity we chose SRM for further study. The same performance as reported below for SRM is possible to obtain with SIM analysis using a column with smaller inner diameter. This is possible since the sensitivity in electrospray is concentration dependent, therefore miniaturization of HPLC equipment is of advantage when high sensitivity is required. During SRM analysis with a 3 mm column eluted at 0.4 ml/min, it is possible to detect all investigated isocyanates with a detection limit (S/N=3, H_{12}MDI) or better (MIC, S/N=16) of 5 pg isocyanate. It is possible to quantify all isocyanates with a quantification limit (S/N=10) of 50 pg isocyanate injected (H_{12}MDI S/N=20, MIC S/N =200). Using 5 µl injections from 2 ml samples this will correspond to a lower quantification limit of 20 ng collected isocyanate.

Gradient elution of eleven common occurring isocyanates quantified with SRM is presented in Fig 3. We achieve a linear detection (correlation coefficient 0.995-0.999) from sample sizes 2 ng - 2 µg. The MDHS 25/3 method requires the detection of 1-140 µg NCO-groups/m^3 from a 15 dm^3 pumped sample. This corresponds to 15 ng - 2.1 µg collected NCO-groups, corresponding to 20 ng - 2.8 µg MIC and 47 ng –6.6 µg H_{12}MDI, respectively. The British short time exposure limit is 20 µg NCO-groups/m^3 that will be collected during 10 min (20 dm^3 of air) sampling period. This corresponds to 500 ng of MIC and 3 µg H_{12}MDI, respectively. The Swedish short time exposure limit is 0.01ppm isocyanate in a sample collected during 5 min (10 dm^3 of air). This corresponds to 200 ng of MIC and 1.0 µg H_{12}MDI, respectively.

The possibility to screen for unknown isocyanates using the m/z 193 ion is demonstrated in Figure 3. It can be seen from the figure that this fragment can be used to identify isocyanate groups. Work is in progress to further study the relationship between analytical responses for monomers and oligomers.

In order to evaluate method reproducibility a sample containing MDI was cleaned up and analyzed six times against six individual calibration curves with and without a chemical analog (2-MP-IPDI) as internal standard (IS). Using the external calibration curve the reproducibility was Aprox 18 %(RSD, n = 18). Using an internal standard the reproducibility was 4% (RSD, n = 18). The determinations were performed within 4 days. Precision, as the standard deviation of 6 injections using the same standard curve, was 3% with IS and 2% without IS.

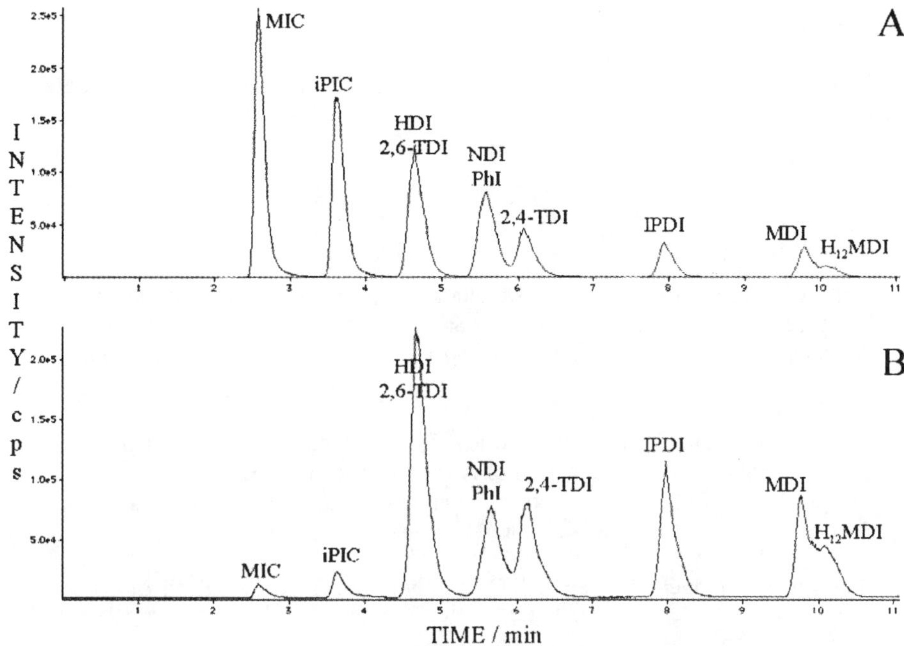

Figure 3 - *The reconstructed ion chromatogram in A is the sum of SRM analysis using the [M+H]$^+$ as parent ion and the m/z 193 as daughter ion. The individual [M+H]$^+$ are MIC m/z 250, iPIC m/z 278, HDI m/z 553, TDI m/z 559, NDI m/z 595, PhI m/z 312, IPDI m/z 607, MDI m/z 635 and H$_{12}$MDI m/z 647. The same standard mixture analyzed with SIM of the [2MP+H]$^+$ fragment m/z 193 demonstrates the possibility to screen for unknown/unexpected isocyanates (B).*

Conclusions

The 2-MP filter method to measure isocyanates in workplace air is an internationally accepted, widespread procedure. We have investigated the conditions for using mass spectrometric detection instead of the combined UV/electrochemical detection. Thereby the selectivity and sensitivity of the method have increased, and the possibility to screen for unknown isocyanates has been added. The sensitivity achieved is improved with the system presented, and can be further enhanced by the use of capillary columns.

Acknowledgment

This work was in part funded by the Swedish National Board for Occupational Safety and Health.

References

[1]   Levin, J. O., Brown, R. H., Ennals, R., Lindahl, R., and Östin, A., "Isocyanates: Measurement Methodology, Exposure and Effects. Report from an International Workshop." *Journal of Environmental Monitoring*, 2000, Vol. 1, No. 6, pp. 18N-20N.

[2]   Streicher, R. P., Reh, C. M., Key-Schwartz, R. J., Schlecht, P. C., Cassinelli, M. E., and O´Connor, P., "Determination of Airborne Isocyanate Exposure: Considerations in Method Selection," *American Industrial Hygiene Association Journal*, 2000, Vol. 61, No. 4, in press.

[3]   Andersson, K., Gudhén, A., Levin, J. O., and Nilsson, C. A., "Analysis of Gaseous Diisocyanates in Air Using Chemosorption Sampling", *Chemosphere,* 1982, Vol. 10, No. 1, pp. 3-10.

[4]   Levin, J. O., "Sampling of Reactive Species. "In *Clean Air at Work - New Trends in Assessment and Measurement for the 1990s*", Brown, R. H., Curtis, M., Saunders, K. J., and Vandendriessche, S. (eds.), Royal Society of Chemistry, Cambridge, 1992, pp. 135-141.

[5]   England, E., Key-Ashwartz, R., Lesage, J., Carlton, G., Streicher, R., and Song, R., "Comparison of Sampling Methods for Monomer and Polyisocyanates of 1,6-Hexamethylene Diisocyanate During Spray Finishing Operations," *Applied Occupational and Environmental Hygiene,* 2000, Vol. 15, No. 6, pp 472-478.

[6]   Health and Safety Executive, "Organic Isocyanates in Air", MDHS 25/3,. Health and Safety Laboratory, UK. 1999.

[7]   White, J., Brown, R. H., and Clench, M. R., "Particle Beam Liquid Chromatography/Mass Spectrometry Analysis of Hazardous Agricultural Chemicals," *Rapid Communications in Mass Spectrometry*, 1997, Vol. 11, pp. 618-623.

Roy J. Rando, [1] Halet G. Poovey, [1] and Dinkar R. Mokadam[1]

Laboratory Comparison of Sampling Methods for Reactive Isocyanate Vapors and Aerosols

---

Reference: Rando, R. J., Poovey, H. G., and Mokadam, D. R., **" Laboratory Comparison of Sampling Methods for Reactive Isocyanate Vapors and Aerosols,"** *Isocyanates: Sampling, Analysis, and Health Effects, ASTM STP 1408*, J. Lesage, I. D. DeGraff, and R. S. Danchik, Eds., American Society for Testing and Materials, West Conshohocken, PA, 2002.

Abstract: Three methods for quantifying test atmospheres of TDI, MDI, and their respective pre-polymers were compared in the laboratory: the modified OSHA 42 sampler, Tulane dichotomous sampler, and the ISO-CHEK™. Grouped samples (both 15-minute and 3-hour sampling periods) were collected from test atmospheres of the monomers ranging from approximately 2 to 20 ppb and of the pre-polymers ranging from 32.2 to 344.2 µg isocyanate/m^3. In these tests, the Tulane sampler consistently yielded the highest results and accurately speciated the isocyanate into vapor and aerosol fractions. The OSHA sampler agreed with the Tulane sampler for MDI but reported lower concentrations of TDI. The ISO-CHEK™ consistently yielded the lowest results for isocyanate monomer and exhibited the highest variability, but it agreed with the Tulane sampler for short-term measurements of isocyanate pre-polymer. While not suitable for personal monitoring, overall the Tulane dichotomous sampler appears to be the most reliable of the devices for either short- or long-term sampling of reactive isocyanate vapors and aerosols.

Keywords: isocyanate, aerosols, diffusional denuder, TDI, MDI, ISO-CHEK™

---

[1] Associate Professor, Research Assistant Professor, and Associate Scientist, respectively, Tulane University, School of Public Health & Tropical Medicine, Department of Environmental Health Sciences, 1430 Tulane Ave. - SL15, New Orleans, LA 70112.

The determination of airborne diisocyanates and total reactive isocyanate group (TRIG) in air is challenging. The isocyanate group is somewhat unstable chemically; it will react with compounds containing labile hydrogen such as alcohols and amines, and it is prone to oligomerization when properly catalyzed. In addition, there is a wide range in physical properties of industrially important isocyanate compounds, particularly in terms of saturated vapor pressure. The saturated vapor concentrations of common isocyanates may range from essentially nil such as that of isocyanate oligomers and pre-polymers, to values of ~5 ppb and ~30 ppm for methylene-bis-phenylisocyanate (MDI) and toluene diisocyanate (TDI) monomers, respectively. This range of vapor pressures can result in the partitioning of TRIG into vapor and particulate phases in the atmosphere. Thus, any technique for TRIG should not only address the issues of chemical stability and the wide variety of possible TRIG forms, but should also speciate the collected TRIG into particulate and vapor fractions, or ensure that collection efficiency is unbiased towards either the aerosol or vapor forms.

With this in mind, the goal of the present work was to evaluate the performance of three sampling devices for collection and measurement of airborne TRIG derived from TDI and MDI. Test atmospheres containing isocyanate in the vapor phase, aerosol phase, and mixtures of both were used to compare the performance of the ISO-CHEK™ sampling system, the Tulane Dichotomous TRIG sampler, and the OSHA 42/47 analytical technique, using a standardized test protocol.

Experimental Methods

ISO-CHEK™ Sampler - The ISO-CHEK[TM] system is based on a technique developed by Lesage, et al.[1,2] and is used in ASTM Standard Test Method for Toluene Diisocyanate in Air, D 5932-96. The sampler consists of a 37-mm filter cassette containing a 5-μm Teflon prefilter backed up by a glass fiber filter. The glass fiber filter is treated with 9-(N-methylamino-methyl)anthracene (MAMA) reagent. Aerosols containing non-volatile isocyanate monomers and oligomers are collected on the prefilter while vapor phase isocyanate monomers pass through and are trapped by the MAMA treated filter. For this work, previously prepared and assembled ISO-CHEK™ samplers were purchased from Omega Specialty Instrument Co. (Chelmsford, MA) and used as received in accordance with the manufacturer's instructions. Sample collection was performed with vacuum pump and critical orifice, or constant-flow personal sampling pumps with a nominal flow rate of 1 L/min. Samples were collected in the closed-face mode for all test atmospheres; in addition, a full set of ISO-CHEK™ samples was collected in the open face mode (cassette top removed) for the TDI-monomer test atmospheres. In the closed-face mode, the sample inlet diameter was 4 mm.

After collection, the Teflon pre-filter was immediately removed from the sampler and desorbed in 5 mL of a solution of 0.1 mg / mL 1-(2-methoxy-phenyl) piperazine (MOPIP) in toluene with sonication for 10 minutes. The samples were then evaporated to dryness under a stream of nitrogen and then were reconstituted with 1.0 mL of 0.5 % v/v acetic anhydride in acetonitrile solution.

Chromatographic analysis of the MOPIP-derivatized samples and standards was performed with detection using a Perkin Elmer Model LC90 UV detector set at a wavelength of 242 nm. An Alcott model 738R autosampler injected 20 µl of the samples. Samples were analyzed on a Supelcosil LC-18-DB 5µm particle size, 4.6 mm i.d. by 25 cm long (Supelco, Belafonte, PA). Mobile phase consisted of a mixture of 65 % acetonitrile and 35 % buffer solution (7.5 g of sodium acetate in 50 / 50 mixture of water and methanol, adjusted to pH 6.0 with acetic acid).

The back-up filter was desorbed with 2.0 mL of a mixture of triethylammonium phosphate buffer, acetonitrile, and dimethylformamide. Chromatographic analysis of these samples and MAMA-urea standards was performed with detection by fluorescence with excitation at 245 nm and emission at 414 nm, and by ultraviolet absorption at 245 nm and 370 nm. Autosampler injected 20 µl of the samples. Samples were analyzed on a Supelcosil LC-8-DB column, 5 µm particle size, 4.6 mm i.d. by 5 cm long. The mobile phase consisted of a mixture of 60% acetonitrile and 40% aqueous triethylammonium phosphate buffer (3% triethylamine in water, adjusted to pH 3.0 with phosphoric acid).

Chromatograms were screened for presence of TRIG-derived peaks by comparison to the appropriate parent monomer standard. The criteria for classification of a peak as being a TRIG-containing compound was a detector response ratio for UV absorbance (245 nm/370 nm) within ± 20% of that for the monomer standard with confirmation by fluorescence response[3,4]. Quantitation of TRIG was determined in comparison to the UV response of the parent monomer standard. Calibration of detector response for quantitation of TRIG in these compounds used conversion factors based on two moles TRIG / mole of diisocyanate monomer.

The Tulane Dichotomous Sampler[5,6] - The dichotomous sampler components were obtained from University Research Glassware (Model 2000, URG, Carrboro, North Carolina). The inlet to the device was an aluminum cyclone with a 14-mm inlet designed to provide separation of the respirable fraction of sampled aerosol. The cyclone was followed by an annular diffusional denuder section, consisting of inner and outer glass cylinders with an annular spacing of 0.1 cm in between. The outer diameter of the denuder tube was 2.6 cm, and the length was 24 cm. The final stage of the sampler was a 37-mm Teflon filter holder containing a treated glass fiber filter. The denuder walls and backup filter were coated with a mixture of MAMA reagent (1 mg) and tributyl-phosphate (20 mg). The dichotomous sampler was operated at a nominal flow rate of 2 L/min.

Immediately after collection, the cyclone inlet was washed with 2.0 mL of a solution of MAMA in dimethyl sulfoxide (DMSO). The denuder and filter were then desorbed with 2.0 mL DMSO, and the cyclone, denuder, and filter samples separately analyzed by HPLC. The analytical conditions and protocol were the same as that used for analysis of the MAMA-treated filter samples from the ISO-CHEK™, as described above.

The OSHA Sampler - A limitation of the OSHA Method 42/47 is that it only identifies and quantitates the isocyanate monomers. It has been reported that the OSHA method may underestimate isocyanate in aerosol form or when sampling for extended periods [7]. It has been suggested that additional 1-(2-pyridyl) piperazine (PYP) be added to the filter (up to 1 mg, in comparison to OSHA's suggested value of 0.1 mg) [8]. The OSHA method 42/47 sampler used in this work was a 13-mm glass fiber filter treated with approximately 0.3 mg of PYP. For sample collection, the treated filter was placed into a polypropylene Swinney cassette with a 4–mm inlet and sample collected at a nominal flow rate of 1 L/min.

After collection, the isocyanate-PYP derivatives were desorbed with 2.0 mL of a 90/10 v/v acetonitrile and DMSO solution with sonication for 10 minutes. Chromatographic analysis of the PYP-derivatized samples and standards was performed with detection by fluorescence with excitation at 240 nm and emission at 370 nm, and by ultraviolet absorption at two wavelengths, 254 nm and 313 nm. Twenty microliters of the samples were injected by autosampler. Samples were analyzed on a Supelcosil LC-8-DB column, 5-µm particle size, 4.6 mm i.d. by 25 cm long. Mobile phase consisted of a mixture of 37.5 % acetonitrile and 62.5 % buffer solution (0.01 M ammonium acetate in water adjusted to pH 6.0 with acetic acid) for TDI or 50/50 acetonitrile/buffer for MDI.

General Testing Protocol - Test atmospheres of various isocyanate materials were generated in the laboratory and simultaneously sampled with the ISO-CHEK™ sampler, the modified OSHA Method 42/47 sampler, and the Tulane dichotomous sampler. The specific isocyanate materials used in these laboratory evaluations were as follows:

- 50% 2,4-TDI / 50% 2,6-TDI: The pure 2,4- and 2,6-isomers of TDI were purchased from Aldrich Chemical Co.
- MDI: MDI (98%) was obtained from Aldrich Chemical Co.
- PMPPI: PMPPI (poly-methlyene-poly-phenylene isocyanate) was a mixture of about 49% MDI monomer and 51% MDI oligomers. It was obtained from Aldrich Chemical Co.
- Rexthane™: Rexthane™ was a moisture cure polyurethane varnish containing approximately 2% TDI monomer, polyurethane prepolymers (polyhydric alcohol-TDI adduct with 0.8% free isocyanate group) and xylene. It was manufactured by Sherwin Williams Co. and purchased from a local Sherwin Williams retail outlet.

For the test atmospheres described above, both short-term (15 minute) and long-term (3 hour) sampling periods were evaluated. For the isocyanate monomers, short-term samples were collected at concentration multiples of the PEL (20 ppb). Long-term samples were collected at the TLV for TDI (5 ppb) and at the TLV (5 ppb) and PEL (20 ppb) for MDI. For the oligomer aerosol test atmospheres, short and long-term samplings were conducted at target concentrations of approximately 0.5 mg/m^3 and 0.1 mg/m^3, respectively. For each test atmosphere, 6 samples were collected for each of the sampler types.

Production of Test Atmospheres - Aerosol test atmospheres of PMPPI and

Rexthane[TM] were generated with a Devilbiss Model 40 glass nebulizer. Test solution was continuously fed into the nebulizer with a syringe pump. For the short term PMPPI atmospheres a 2.5% solution of PMPPI in acetone was injected at a rate of 350 μL/min with a nitrogen flow of 6 L/min through the nebulizer. For the long term atmospheres, a 0.2 % solution was injected at 350 μL/min with a nitrogen flow of 7 L/min. The short term TDI polymer atmosphere was generated by nebulizing a 1:8 Rexthane[TM] in reducer solution at 350 μL/min with a nitrogen flow of 6 L/min. The long term TDI polymer atmospheres were generated by nebulizing a 1:20 Rexthane[TM] in reducer solution at 350 μL/min with a nitrogen flow of 5 L/min. The estimated mass median diameter and geometric standard deviation of the prepolymer aerosols were approximately 1.5 μm and 1.8, respectively, based on the reported output characteristics of this nebulizer [9] and the dilution ratio of isocyanate prepolymer to solvent.

The polymer aerosols were produced in an aerosol test chamber (137 cm x 31 cm x 31 cm) operated under positive pressure at a flow rate of about 2800 L/min, resulting in an average flow velocity of 51 cm/s (100 ft/min) in the sampling cross-section.[6] A series of perforated plate diffusers ensured mixing of aerosol and dilution air. The aerosol atmosphere passed through a honeycomb flow straightener (tubular cells of 28-mm diameter and 155-mm length) before entering the sampling zone. Samplers were placed side-by-side at the same vertical level inside the chamber and their actual positions in the sampling cross-section were randomized from run to run.

Test atmospheres of TDI and MDI monomers were produced in a laminar flow test chamber [5]. The chamber was a horizontal laminar flow cabinet with dimensions of 2.4 m x 1.2 m x 1.8 m (8 ft. x 4 ft. x 6 ft) and was constructed from stainless steel and glass. Dilution flow through the chamber varied between 2.8 m^3/min (99 cfm) and 9.0 m^3/min (317 cfm) with a resulting flow velocity of about 1.2 m/min (4.1 ft/min) to 4.0 m/min (13.2 ft/min).

Vapor atmospheres of TDI were generated by a simple saturation technique. The liquid isocyanate was placed in a fritted glass bubbler (Ace Glass No. 7430) and dry nitrogen was bubbled through, resulting in a saturated stream which was then fed into the chamber. A glass fiber filter was placed in line between the generator and the chamber to prevent induction of any aerosolized TDI into the chamber. The target concentration of the test atmosphere was achieved by adjustment of the flow rates of the isocyanate-saturated nitrogen and of the dilution air through the chamber. Nitrogen flow rates ranged from 1.2 to 5.6 L/min.

Mixed atmospheres of vapor and condensation aerosol of MDI were generated by a flash evaporation technique [5]. The isocyanate was metered to a heated, nitrogen-flushed generator by a syringe pump. The generator temperature was controlled at approximately 250°C. The generator outlet line to the injection port on the chamber was maintained at a temperature of 160°C. For generation of MDI, a solution of 1% MDI in acetone was used with a nitrogen flow of 7.5 L/min. Target concentrations were attained by adjusting the syringe pump injection rate. Injection rates ranged from 40 to 300 μL/min. The condensation aerosol produced has a count median diameter of 1.1 μm with a geometric standard deviation of 1.2 [5].

Results

Temperature and relative humidity ranged from 22 to 26°C and 42 to 63%, respectively, across the various experiments. OSHA samples were used in all the test atmospheres examined; however, isocyanate monomer in the OSHA samples from the PMPPI and Rexthane[TM] atmospheres could not be determined because of the presence of major interfering peaks in the sample chromatograms.

MDI Monomer Atmospheres

Short Term Sampling Results - Fifteen-minute samples from MDI atmospheres were collected in groups of three of each sampler type. Eight test atmospheres were sampled and ranged from 24.5 to 449 $\mu g/m^3$ (2.9 to 42.3 ppb) MDI, on average, according to the OSHA sampler. Linear regression of the results from the Tulane Dichotomous sampler and the ISO-CHEK[TM] sampler against the OSHA sampler yielded the following regression lines (Figure 1):

$$Tulane = 1.00\,OSHA + 0.4, \ r^2 = 0.999; \quad Isochek = 0.88\,OSHA - 11.4, \ r^2 = 0.942$$

The Tulane and OSHA samplers provided nearly identical results across the test

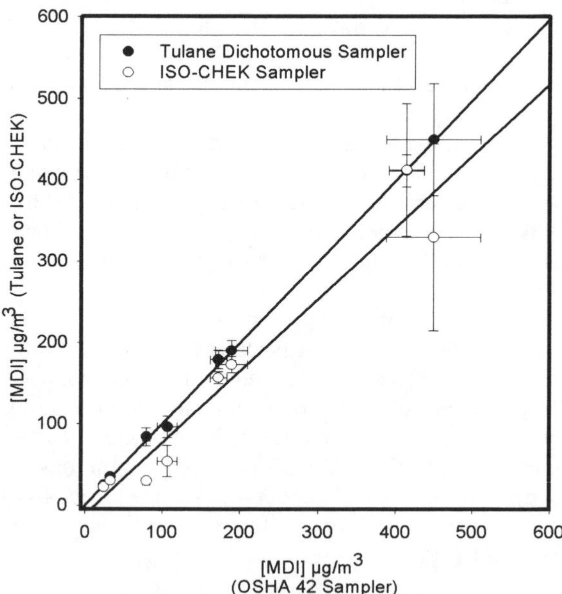

Figure 1 - *Comparison of Sampler Performance for MDI Monomer Atmospheres - Short Term (15-minute) Samples*

atmospheres. The ISO-CHEK[TM] reported MDI concentrations lower than both the OSHA and Tulane dichotomous samplers. Overall, the ISO-CHEK[TM] values appeared to be approximately 15% lower than the other samplers, on average.

Both the OSHA sampler and the Tulane dichotomous sampler exhibited precision of about 7% RSD (relative standard deviation) which was fairly constant across the concentration range. The ISO-CHEK[TM] sampler exhibited precision which ranged from about 4% RSD to about 35% RSD and which varied unpredictably.
Both the Tulane dichotomous sampler and the ISO-CHEK[TM] sampler reportedly are able to speciate the sample into the vapor and condensed phases. For the Tulane dichotomous sampler, the aerosol fraction of the sample is collected in the cyclone inlet and the back-up filter, whereas in the ISO-CHEK[TM], it is found on the Teflon pre-filter. The measured fraction of MDI in the aerosol phase as a function of the total MDI concentration for these experiments is shown in Figure 2.

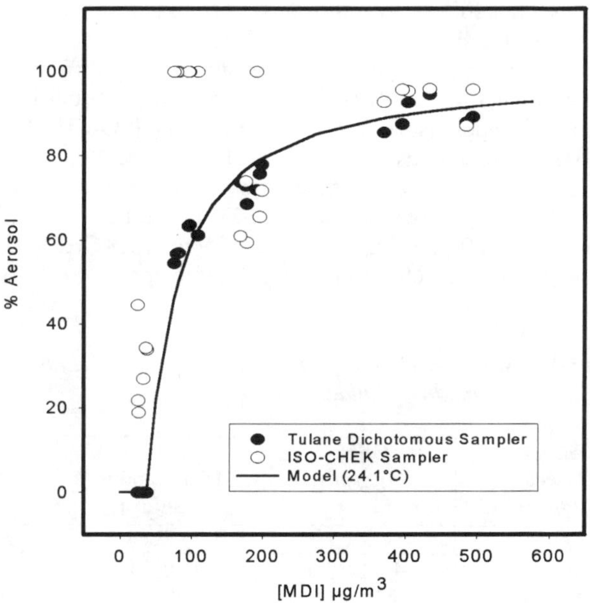

Figure 2 - *Vapor/Aerosol Fractionation of MDI Test Atmospheres: 15-Minute Samples*

Overlaid on the data in Figure 2 is a model based on the saturated vapor concentration of 4,4'-MDI [*10*]. For the average test atmosphere temperature of 24.1°C (range: 22.8 - 26.3°C), the model assumes a saturated vapor concentration of approximately 41 µg/m³ for 4,4'-MDI and has the following form:

$$\text{If } [\textbf{MDI}] \leq 41 \ \mu g/m^3, \text{ then } \% \text{ aero} = 0;$$
$$\text{If } [\textbf{MDI}] > 41 \ \mu g/m^3, \text{ then } \textbf{\% aero} = \{[\textbf{MDI}] - 41\}/[\textbf{MDI}] \times 100$$

Where $[\textbf{MDI}]$ is the concentration of MDI in the test atmosphere, and $\textbf{\% aero}$ is the predicted percentage of MDI present in the aerosol fraction.

The results from the Tulane dichotomous sampler are in very close agreement to that predicted by the model. In contrast, the ISO-CHEK[TM] indicates the presence of about 20 to 45% aerosol below the saturation concentration of 41 $\mu g/m^3$, with varying but increasing percentages above. This suggests that the Teflon pre-filter in the ISO-CHEK[TM] adsorbs significant amounts of MDI vapor, and thus misrepresents the fractionation of MDI into vapor and aerosol.

Long-Term Sampling Results - These samples were collected in groups of three of each type of sampler and at two target concentration levels; 51 $\mu g/m^3$ (5 ppb) and 205 $\mu g/m^3$ (20 ppb). The test atmospheres averaged 25.6°C (range: 24.6 - 26.3°C) and 52% (range: 50 - 55%) relative humidity.

The Tulane and OSHA sampler results were not significantly different (Table 1). The ratio of the Tulane sampler to the OSHA sampler averaged 1.06 and 1.03 at the target levels of 5 ppb and 20 ppb, respectively. In contrast, the ISO-CHEK[TM] sampler under-reported the MDI concentrations, with statistically significant differences between it and the other sampling devices in three of the four experimental runs. For the 5-ppb target level, the ISO-CHEK[TM] reported, on average, 62% of the Tulane sampler and 67% of the OSHA sampler. At the 20-ppb target level, the average ISO-CHEK[TM] response was 67% of the Tulane sampler and 69% of the OSHA sampler.

Table 1 - *Sample Results for MDI Monomer - Long-Term (3-Hour) Samples (mean ± standard deviation)*

Run No.	Target Level ($\mu g/m^3$)	OSHA ($\mu g/m^3$)	Tulane Dichotomous ($\mu g/m^3$)	ISO-CHEK[TM] ($\mu g/m^3$)
*M-L-1	51	54.8 ± 1.5	55.4 ± 4.7	23.7 ± 4.5
M-L-2	51	43.2 ± 2.8	48.0 ± 1.7	38.8 ± 5.3
*M-L-3	205	226 ± 11	229 ± 17	136 ± 23
*M-L-4	205	197 ± 4	206 ± 8	152 ± 15

* *significant differences across sample type ($p < 0.05$) by ANOVA on $\mu g/m^3$ MDI*

As in the short-term sampling results, the precision of the OSHA and Tulane methods in the long-term sampling experiments was comparable and was in the range of about 5% RSD. The precision of the ISO-CHEK[TM] was 14.9% RSD, on average, and ranged from 9.9 to 19%.

TDI Monomer Atmospheres

Short-Term Sampling Results - Fifteen-minute samples were collected from test atmospheres of TDI monomer at four target concentrations. For each target concentration, six experimental runs were done in which one representative of each sampler type was used to collect sample. For each run, two ISO-CHEK^{TM} samples - one in the open-face mode and one in the closed-face mode - were simultaneously collected. The results were compared by a series of linear regression analyses (Figure 3).

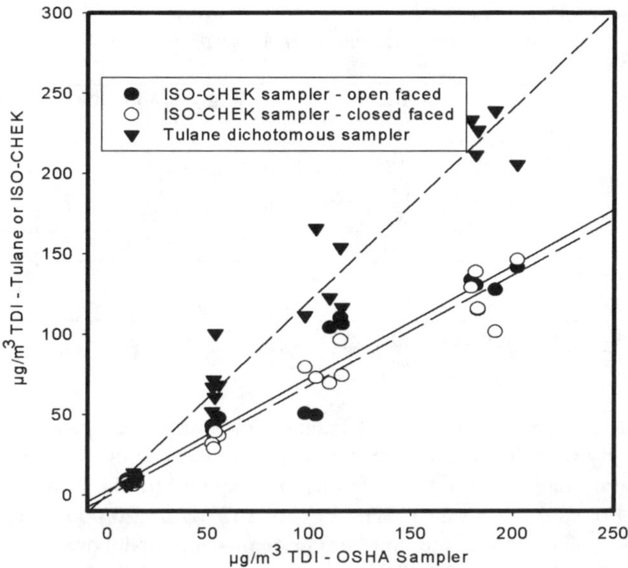

Figure 3 - *Comparison of Sampling Devices for Total TDI Monomer; 15-Minute Sampling Period*

Overall, the OSHA sampler indicated about 20% less than the Tulane sampler, whereas the ISO-CHEK^{TM} underreported by about 45% in comparison to the Tulane sampler. There were apparent differences in the disparity in response for the individual isomers of TDI, and whether ISO-CHEK^{TM} sampling was conducted in the open- or closed-face mode. In order to examine whether these differences were statistically significant, multivariate linear regression analyses were performed. The multivariate regression models included dummy variables for TDI isomer and for the ISO-CHEK^{TM} sampling mode. The models are shown below:

$$[ISO\text{-}CHEK] = \beta_0 + \beta_1\,[Tulane] + \beta_2\,'Mode' + \beta_3\,'Isomer', \text{ and}$$

$$[OSHA] = \beta_4 + \beta_5\,[Tulane] + \beta_6\,'Isomer'$$

where *[ISO-CHEK]*, *[Tulane]*, and *[OSHA]* are the concentrations of TDI monomer reported by the ISO-CHEK^{TM}, Tulane dichotomous, and OSHA 42 samplers, respectively, in units of µg/m^3; *'Mode'* is the dummy variable for ISO-CHEK^{TM} sampling mode, with 0 = closed face and 1 = open face; and *'Isomer'* is the dummy variable for TDI isomer, with 0 = 2,4-TDI and 1= 2,6-TDI.

For the ISO-CHEK^{TM}, the results of this analysis show no statistical dependence of response on the isomer of TDI or on sampling in the closed- versus open-face mode (Table 2). Accordingly, the data indicate that overall, the ISO-CHEK^{TM} reports TDI concentrations that are about 55% of that reported by the Tulane dichotomous sampler.

Table 2 - *Results of Multi-Variate Linear Regression Models for 15-Minute Samples from TDI Monomer Test Atmospheres*

	Coefficient	Regression value	p-value
ISO-CHEK^{TM} v. Tulane n = 88; r^2 = 0.887	β_0	-0.6	0.76
	*β_1	0.55	<0.0001
	β_2	2.25	0.21
	β_3	2.40	0.19
OSHA v. Tulane n = 44; r^2 = 0.953	*β_4	5.2	0.0127
	*β_5	0.79	<0.0001
	*β_6	-7.05	0.0035

*statistically significant at α = 0.05

In comparing the OSHA sampler and Tulane dichotomous sampler, the model indicates statistically significant differences in response between the isomers of TDI. However, the overall magnitude of the difference in response for the isomers is relatively small. For example, at the OSHA PEL of 142 µg/m^3 (20 ppb) as reported by the Tulane dichotomous sampler, the multivariate regression model predicts OSHA sampler values of 118 µg/m^3 for 2,4-TDI, and 111 µg/m^3 for 2,6-TDI.

Long-Term Sampling Results - Three-hour sampling of TDI monomer test atmospheres was performed at a target concentration of 36 µg/m^3 (5 ppb) total TDI. Six experimental runs were done using one sampler of each type. Temperature and relative humidity of the test atmospheres ranged from 22.8°C to 23.6°C and 60% to 65%, respectively.

An analysis of variance (ANOVA) of the total TDI monomer data (Table 3) showed statistically significant differences in response across the sampler types (p < 0.0001). Pair-wise comparisons using the Student-Newman-Keuls method (SNK) indicated that there were statistically significant differences between the Tulane dichotomous sampler and all the rest of the sampler types, between the OSHA sampler and the ISO-CHEK^{TM} sampler in the closed-face mode, but not between the OSHA sampler and the open-face ISO-CHEK^{TM}, nor between the two ISO-CHEK^{TM} sampling modes. In comparison to the Tulane dichotomous sampler, the average OSHA response was 63%, whereas for the ISO-CHEK[TM] it was 38% and 52% for the closed- and open-face sampling modes, respectively.

The data for total TDI monomer was derived from test atmospheres that contained, on average, 43% 2,4-TDI and 57% 2,6-TDI. A two-way ANOVA was performed on the data, with isomer and sampler type as the treatment variables. After accounting for the differences in concentrations of the isomers, there were statistically significant differences in the performance of the samplers ($p < 0.0001$) but there was no statistically significant interaction between isomer and sampler type ($p = 0.25$).

Table 3 - *Results of 3-Hour Samples of TDI Monomer Test Atmospheres:(Total TDI)*

Sampler	Mean ± s.d. ($\mu g/m^3$)
OSHA	22.5 ± 5.8
Tulane dichotomous	35.8 ± 6.8
ISO-CHEK[TM] - closed face	13.5 ± 4.1
ISO-CHEK[TM] - open face	18.6 ± 3.5

The SNK pair-wise comparisons procedure indicated that there were statistically significant differences in response between the Tulane dichotomous sampler and all the other sampler types, and between the OSHA sampler and the closed-face ISO-CHEK[TM] sampler, but not the open-face ISO-CHEK[TM]. These results are similar to that seen when analyzing response for total TDI. However, after accounting for the effect of TDI isomer, there was a statistically significant difference in response between the open- and closed-face ISO-CHEK[TM] sampling modes ($p < 0.05$). For total TDI, the ratio of open- to closed-face response was an average of 1.38, while for the isomers, the average ratios were 1.38 and 1.39 for 2,4-TDI and 2,6-TDI, respectively.

PMPPI Atmospheres

Six samples of both the Tulane dichotomous sampler and the ISO-CHEK[TM] sampler were collected under each of 2 sampling regimens: 15-minute samples of PMPPI atmospheres containing an average of 344 $\mu g/m^3$ TRIG, and 3-hour samples of PMPPI atmospheres containing an average of 32 $\mu g/m^3$ TRIG. For each sampling regimen, 3 experimental runs were performed in which 2 pairs of each sampler type were simultaneously collected.

Short-Term Sampling Results - The temperature and relative humidity of the 15-minute test atmospheres of PMPPI were 22.5°C and 63%, respectively. The concentrations of TRIG and MDI in these test atmospheres of PMPPI averaged 344 and 589 $\mu g/m^3$, respectively, as indicated by the Tulane dichotomous sampler (Table 4). The equivalent concentration of the MDI in terms of TRIG would be 198 $\mu g/m^3$; thus MDI monomer constituted approximately 58% of the isocyanate present in the test atmosphere.

The results from the ISO-CHEK[TM] and Tulane dichotomous samplers agreed for TRIG in the 15-minute samples. On average, the ratio of ISO-CHEK[TM] to Tulane dichotomous sampler was 0.98 and there was no statistically significant difference between the samplers when analyzed by a 2-way ANOVA procedure.

In contrast, the ISO-CHEK[TM] consistently reported lower amounts of MDI monomer in comparison to the Tulane sampler. On average, the ratio of ISO-CHEK[TM] to Tulane dichotomous sampler was 0.83, and there was a statistically significant difference between the sampler types after accounting for differences in the experimental runs by a 2-way ANOVA (p = 0.008). This result was also in agreement with that from the short-term sampling of MDI monomer atmospheres in which the average ratio was approximately 0.85.

Table 4 - *Results of 15-Minute Samples of PMPPI Atmospheres*

Run No.	Mean [S.D.] ($\mu g/m^3$)				ISO-CHEK[TM]/ Dichotomous Sampler		P-value* (Sampler type)	
	Dichotomous Sampler		ISO-CHEK[TM]					
	TRIG	MDI	TRIG	MDI	TRIG	MDI	TRIG	MDI
P-S-9	172 [20]	361 [54]	174 [14]	258 [7]	1.01	0.71		
P-S-10	477 [31]	751 [47]	461 [29]	686 [23]	0.97	0.91	0.57	0.008
P-S-11	384 [32]	656 [25]	367 [41]	571 [46]	0.96	0.87		
				Average =	0.98	0.83		

* 2-Way ANOVA (experiment & sampler type)

According to the Tulane dichotomous sampler, the MDI monomer in the 15-minute PMPPI atmosphere samples was present in the aerosol phase at a proportion of 91.2%, on average, whereas the ISO-CHEK[TM] sampler indicated 95.3% of MDI in the aerosol phase, on average. At a temperature of 22.5°C and an average concentration of 589 $\mu g/m^3$, the MDI aerosolization model would predict an aerosol proportion of 95%, based on an equivalent saturated vapor concentration of about 30 $\mu g/m^3$ for 4,4'-MDI at the test temperature.

Long-Term Sampling Results - The temperature and relative humidity of the 3-hour test atmospheres of PMPPI were 22.4°C and 62%, respectively. The concentrations of TRIG and MDI in these test atmospheres of PMPPI averaged 32 and 50 $\mu g/m^3$, respectively, as indicated by the Tulane dichotomous sampler. Again, the equivalent concentration of the MDI in terms of TRIG would be 17 $\mu g/m^3$, so that the MDI monomer constituted approximately 53% of the isocyanate present in these test atmospheres.

On average, the ratios of ISO-CHEK[TM] to Tulane dichotomous sampler for the 3-hour samples of PMPPI test atmosphere were 0.68 and 0.64, for TRIG and MDI monomer, respectively (Table 5). The differences were statistically significant for both isocyanate species when analyzed by a 2-way ANOVA that accounted for differences in concentration between the experimental runs. The observed difference in response was essentially the same for both TRIG and MDI in the PMPPI atmospheres and furthermore, were comparable to the results seen for the 3-hour sampling of MDI monomer atmospheres as previously discussed (see Table 1).

Table 5 - *Results of 3-Hour Samples of PMPPI Atmospheres*

Run No.	Mean [S.D.] ($\mu g/m^3$)				ISO-CHEK[TM]/ Dichotomous Sampler		P-value* (Sampler type)	
	Dichotomous Sampler		ISO-CHEK					
	TRIG	MDI	TRIG	MDI	TRIG	MDI	TRIG	MDI
P-L-12	33.6 [1.2]	51.6 [0.8]	21.9 [3.9]	30.3 [8.0]	0.65	0.59		
P-L-13	31.1 [4.0]	44.3 [2.2]	23.4 [2.6]	32.8 [13.3]	0.75	0.74	0.0006	0.003
P-L-14	31.9 [1.8]	53.8 [3.0]	20.0 [1.5]	31.0 [3.6]	0.63	0.58		
				Average	0.68	0.64		

*2-Way ANOVA (experiment & sampler type)

For the 3-hour test atmospheres for PMPPI, the MDI aerosolization model predicts an aerosol proportion of 40%, based on a saturated vapor concentration of about 30 $\mu g/m^3$ for 4,4'-MDI at the test temperature and a test atmosphere concentration of 50 $\mu g/m^3$. In comparison, the Tulane dichotomous sampler indicated an average aerosol fraction of 59% of MDI. In contrast, the ISO-CHEK[TM] sampler reported MDI present as aerosol at a proportion of 90%, on average. The difference in total MDI reported by the two devices appears to be driven primarily by the respective difference in the observed MDI vapor levels. For example, in comparing only the apparent levels of MDI aerosol, the devices are very similar with the Tulane dichotomous sampler indicating an overall mean of 26.1 ± 3.7 $\mu g/m^3$, whereas the ISO-CHEK[TM] indicates 28.8 ± 7.3 $\mu g/m^3$.

Rexthane[TM] Atmospheres

Six samples of both the Tulane dichotomous sampler and the ISO-CHEK[TM] sampler were collected under each of 2 sampling regimens: 15-minute samples of Rexthane[TM] atmospheres containing an average of 202 $\mu g/m^3$ TRIG, and 3-hour samples of Rexthane[TM] atmospheres containing an average of 31 $\mu g/m^3$ TRIG. For each sampling regimen, 3 experimental runs were performed in which 2 pairs of each sampler type were simultaneously collected.

Short-Term Sampling Results - The temperature and relative humidity of the 15-minute test atmospheres of Rexthane[TM] were 24.4°C and 54%, respectively. The concentrations of TRIG and TDI in these test atmospheres averaged 202 and 62.3 $\mu g/m^3$, respectively, as indicated by the Tulane dichotomous sampler. The TDI monomer was composed of 15.5 $\mu g/m^3$ (25%) 2,4-TDI and 46.8 $\mu g/m^3$ (75%) 2,6-TDI, on average. In terms of TRIG, the concentration of 62.3 $\mu g/m^3$ TDI is equal to 30 $\mu g/m^3$; thus TDI monomer constituted approximately 15% of the isocyanate present.

Table 6 - *Results of 15-Minute Samples of Rexthane Atmospheres*

Run No.	Mean ±[S.D.] ($\mu g/m^3$)						ISO-CHEK[TM]/ Dichotomous Sampler			P-value* (Sampler type)		
	Dichotomous Sampler			ISO-CHEK[TM]								
	TRI G	2,4- TDI	2,6- TDI	TRI G	2,4- TDI	2,6- TDI	TRI G	2,4- TDI	2,6- TDI	TRI G	2,4- TDI	2,6- TDI
RS-15	214 [25]	18.0 [1.8]	51.4 [7.0]	202 [27]	nd	14.9 [1.3]	0.95	---	0.29			
RS-16	188 [17]	13.6 [3.8]	40.4 [10.9]	169 [2.4]	nd	16.4 [3.7]	0.90	---	0.41	0.10	---	<0.01
RS-17	202 [9.6]	14.9 [0.6]	48.7 [2.2]	172 [11]	nd	15.2 [1.8]	0.85	---	0.31			
						Average =	0.90	---	0.34			

*2-Way ANOVA (experiment & sampler type)
nd: less than limit of detection (~2.5 $\mu g/m^3$ for vapor; ~7 $\mu g/m^3$ for aerosol)

The results indicated a consistently lower response by the ISO-CHEK[TM]. On average, the ratio of ISO-CHEK[TM] to Tulane dichotomous sampler was 0.9; however, the difference between the two sampling devices was not statistically significant when analyzed by a 2-way ANOVA (Table 6).

In contrast, the ISO-CHEK[TM] consistently reported much lower amounts of TDI monomer in comparison to the Tulane sampler. The ISO-CHEK[TM] sampler detected no 2,4-TDI in the samples whereas the Tulane dichotomous sampler saw an average of 15.5 $\mu g/m^3$ (2.2 ppb). For the 2,6-isomer, the average ratio of ISO-CHEK[TM] to Tulane sampler was 0.34, and there was a statistically significant difference ($p < 0.0001$) between the sampler types after accounting for differences in the experimental runs.

According to the Tulane dichotomous sampler, the 2,4-TDI monomer in the 15-minute Rexthane atmosphere samples was present in the vapor phase at a proportion of $40 \pm 7\%$, on average, which was equivalent to a vapor concentration of 6 $\mu g/m^3$ (0.9 ppb) and an aerosol concentration of 9 $\mu g/m^3$ (1.3 ppb). The Tulane sampler indicated that $61 \pm 4\%$ of 2,6-TDI was in the vapor phase, or 29 $\mu g/m^3$ (4 ppb), on average. All of the 2,6-isomer measured by the ISO-CHEK™ sampler was recovered from the treated filter, indicating isocyanate in the vapor phase. Comparing only the vapor phase 2,6-TDI concentrations reported by the two devices, the ISO-CHEK™ still underreported TDI in comparison to the Tulane dichotomous sampler by an average of 46% (ratio of ISO-CHEK™:Tulane = 0.54).

Long-Term Sampling Results - The temperature and relative humidity of the 3-hour test atmospheres were 24.4°C and 49%, respectively. The concentrations of TRIG and TDI in these test atmospheres averaged 31 and 5.2 $\mu g/m^3$, respectively, as indicated by the Tulane dichotomous sampler. Again, the equivalent concentration of the TDI in terms of TRIG would be 2.5 $\mu g/m^3$, so that TDI monomer constituted approximately 8% of the isocyanate present in these test atmospheres. On average, the 2,4-isomer accounted for 23% of the TDI monomer.

The ratio of ISO-CHEK™ to Tulane dichotomous sampler was 0.35 for TRIG (Table 7). The differences between the ISO-CHEK™ and the Tulane dichotomous sampler were statistically significant when analyzed by a 2-way ANOVA which accounted for differences in concentration between the experimental runs.

2,4-TDI was not detected in any of the 3-hour ISO-CHEK™ samples taken from the Rexthane™ test atmospheres. For these experiments, the Tulane dichotomous sampler reported an average of 1.2 $\mu g/m^3$, of which $40 \pm 8\%$ was present in the vapor phase, equivalent to 0.47 $\mu g/m^3$ (0.07 ppb). The ISO-CHEK™ sampler indicated an average of 2.7 $\mu g/m^3$ of 2,6-TDI in the 3-hour Rexthane™ samples, all of which was observed in the vapor phase. The Tulane dichotomous sampler reported an average of 4.0 $\mu g/m^3$ 2,6-TDI, with 66% or 2.6 $\mu g/m^3$ (0.35 ppb) being in the vapor phase. For total 2,6-TDI, the differences between the Tulane dichotomous and ISO-CHEK™ samplers was statistically significant by 2-way ANOVA.

Table 7 - *Results of 3-Hour Samples of Rexthane Atmospheres*

Run No.	Mean [S.D.] ($\mu g/m^3$)						ISO-CHEK™/ Dichotomous Sampler			P-value* (Sampler type)		
	Dichotomous Sampler			ISO-CHEK™								
	TRIG	2,4-TDI	2,6-TDI	TRIG	2,4-TDI	2,6-TDI	TRIG	2,4-TDI	2,6-TDI	TRIG	2,4-TDI	2,6-TDI
RL-18	30.1 [0.2]	1.0 [0.6]	3.5 [1.2]	8.3 [2.4]	nd	3.8 [1.4]	0.28	---	1.09			
RL-19	27.6 [1.7]	0.9 [0.4]	3.5 [0.3]	10.7 [2.7]	nd	1.9 [0.2]	0.39	---	0.54	<0.01	---	<0.05
RL-20	34.5 [5.3]	1.7 [0.1]	5.0 [0.1]	13.4 [9.1]	nd	2.6 [0.6]	0.39	---	0.52			
						Average =	0.35	---	0.72			

* 2-Way ANOVA (experiment & sampler type)
nd: less than limit of detection (~0.2 $\mu g/m^3$ vapor; ~0.6 $\mu g/m^3$ aerosol)

Summary and Conclusions

The study results are summarized in Table 8. The ISO-CHEK[TM] sampler appears to significantly underestimate isocyanate monomer concentrations and inaccurately apportions them into vapor and aerosol phases. Long-term sampling of aerosol isocyanates with the ISO-CHEK[TM] is especially problematic, as they appear to undergo significant deterioration on the untreated pre-filter during the sampling period. The manufacturer of the ISO-CHEK[TM] recommends using the device for short-term sampling only and the latter result was expected. However, the deficiency in performance under short-term sampling regimens was not anticipated. It is unclear whether these results represent an inherent defect in the design of the device, such as an insufficient loading of MAMA reagent on the back-up filter, or whether there was a transient problem with the sample lots used in this work. Further testing is warranted to investigate this problem.

The OSHA sampler agreed closely with the Tulane dichotomous sampler for MDI monomer but under-reported TDI monomer by about 20 to 40% depending on the duration of sampling. Similar results have been reported by others and the performance of the OSHA sampler could probably have been improved by further increasing the amount of PYP reagent on the filter [8], and using a larger diameter filter cassette to reduce sampling velocity through the device [7].

Table 8 - *Summary of the Study Results*

	Average ratio: ISO-CHEK[TM]/Tulane		Average Ratio: OSHA/Tulane	
	15-minute	3-hour	15-minute	3-hour
TDI	0.55	0.38	0.83	0.63
MDI	0.85	0.64	1.00	0.96
Rexthane[TM]	0.90 (TRIG) <0.34 (TDI)	0.35 (TRIG) <0.72 (TDI)	---	---
PMPPI	0.98 (TRIG) 0.83 (MDI)	0.68 (TRIG) 0.64 (MDI)	---	---

Acknowledgment

This work was supported by the International Isocyanate Institute.

References

[1]   Lesage, J., Goyer, N., Desjardins, F., Vincent, J. Y., and Perrault, G., "Worker's Exposure To Isocyanates," *American Industrial Hygiene Association Journal*, Vol. 53, 1992, pp. 146-153.

[2]   Lesage, J. and Perrault, G., U.S. Patent 4,961,916. 9 Oct. 1990.

[3]   Rando, R. J., Poovey, H. G., Lefante, J. J., and Esmundo, F. R., "Evaluation Of 9-Methylamino-Methylanthracene As A Chemical Label For Total Reactive Isocyanate Group: A Comparison Of Mono- And Di-Isocyanate Monomers," *Journal of Liquid Chromatography*, Vol. 16, 1993, pp. 3977-3996.

[4]   Rando, R. J., Poovey, H. G. and Gibson, R. A., "Evaluation Of 9-Methylamino-Methylanthracene As A Chemical Label For Total Reactive Isocyanates Group: Application To Isocyanate Oligomers, Polyurethane Precursors, And Phosgene," *Journal of Liquid Chromatography*, Vol. 18, 1995, pp. 2743-2763.

[5]   Rando, R. J., Poovey, H. G., "Dichotomous Sampling Of Vapor And Aerosol Of Methylene-Bis-(Phenylisocyanate) [MDI] With An Annular Diffusional Denuder," *American Industrial Hygiene Association Journal*, Vol. 55, 1994, pp. 716-721.

[6]   Rando, R. J., Poovey, H. G., "Development And Application Of A Dichotomous Vapor/Aerosol Sampler For HDI-Derived Total Reactive Isocyanate Group," *American Industrial Hygiene Association Journal*, Vol. 60, 1999, pp. 737-746.

[7]   Podolak, G. E., Cassidy, R. A., Esposito, G. G., and Kippenberger, D. J., "Collection and Analysis of Airborne Hexamethylene Diisocyanate by a Modified OSHA Method," *Sampling and Calibration for Atmospheric Measurements, ASTM STP 957*, J. K. Taylor, Ed., American Society for Testing and Materials, West Conshohocken, PA, 1987, pp. 203-214.

[8]   Dharmarajan, V., Lingg, R. D., Booth, K. S., and Hackathorn, D. R., "Recent Developments in the Sampling and Analysis of Isocyanates in Air," *Sampling and Calibration for Atmospheric Measurements, ASTM STP 957*, J. K. Taylor, Ed., American Society for Testing and Materials, West Conshohocken, PA, 1987, pp. 190-202.

[9]   Cheng, Y. S., and Chen B. T., "Aerosol Sampler Calibration," *Air Sampling Instruments, 8th ed.*, B. S. Cohen and S. V. Hering, Eds., American Conference of Governmental Industrial Hygienists, Cincinnati, OH, 1995, p. 174.

[10] Brochhagen, F. K., Shal, H. P., "Diphenylmethane Diisocyanate: The Concentration Of Its Saturated Vapor," *American Industrial Hygiene Association Journal*, Vol. 47, 1986, pp. 225-228.

Mary Jo Reilly,[1] Kenneth D. Rosenman,[1] and John H. Peck[2]

Work-Related Asthma from Exposure to Isocyanate Levels Below the Michigan OSHA Permissible Exposure Limit

---

Reference: Reilly, M. J., Rosenman, K. D., and Peck, J. H., **"Work-Related Asthma from Exposure to Isocyanate Levels Below the Michigan OSHA Permissible Exposure Limit,"** *Isocyanates: Sampling, Analysis, and Health Effects, ASTM STP 1408*, J. Lesage, I. D. DeGraff, and R. S. Danchik, Eds., American Society for Testing and Materials, West Conshohocken, PA, 2002.

Abstract: This paper examines the characteristics of 261 work-related asthma (WRA) cases exposed to isocyanates reported to an occupational disease surveillance system in Michigan from 1988-1998, and reviews Michigan Occupational Safety and Health Act (OSHA) inspections at 42 of the facilities where they worked. After October of 1993 when the Michigan OSHA program implemented a newer sampling methodology for isocyanates, 42 inspections were conducted in relation to the WRA cases reported. Samples for isocyanates were not collected in one facility. Isocyanate air levels at 40 of the 41 companies where measurements were taken revealed exposures <0.005 parts per million (ppm), as a time-weighted average (TWA). Sampling for isocyanates at one company revealed a level of 0.005 ppm for TDI (TWA).

At 36 of the 42 inspections, similarly exposed co-workers as the index cases completed a breathing symptom questionnaire. Although non-significant, companies were more likely to have co-workers indicate breathing symptoms where the index case reported exposure to one or more isocyanate spills (11 of 13 companies with spills vs. 15 of 23 companies without spills; OR 2.93, 95% CL 0.43-34), and a higher average percent of symptomatic co-workers compared to the companies where the index case reported no spills (23% vs. 16%; OR 1.42, 95% CL 0.99-2.03). Again, although non-significant, there were more MDI-using companies in which at least one co-worker reported breathing problems than TDI or HDI-users (83% vs. 67% vs. 56%; chi-square 2.49, p=0.29). MDI-using companies had a higher average percentage of symptomatic co-

---

[1] Epidemiologist and Professor of Medicine, respectively, Michigan State University, Department of Medicine, 117 West Fee Hall, East Lansing, MI 48824.

[2] Chief, Occupational Health Division, Michigan Department of Consumer and Industry Services, Bureau of Safety and Regulation, PO Box 30649, Lansing, MI 48909.

workers than TDI-users and HDI-users (23% vs. 15% vs. 14%; chi-square 9.92, p=0.007).

Michigan workers are exposed to isocyanates below permissible exposure limits yet continue to develop WRA. Spills may account for some but not all of these cases. Despite the lower volatility of MDI, co-workers with exposure to MDI were more likely to have respiratory symptoms than co-workers exposed to TDI or HDI. The majority of these 42 isocyanate-using companies (72%) had no medical surveillance program to monitor for worker sensitization. Compliance with OSHA laws, or "being within permissible exposure limits " will not guarantee the prevention of WRA. Effective engineering controls, established spill clean-up procedures, a comprehensive hazard communication program, and a medical surveillance program to identify newly sensitized workers for prompt removal from exposure may help to prevent isocyanate-induced WRA. Further work is needed to determine the relative effectiveness of each of these components in preventing isocyanate-exposed workers from developing asthma.

Keywords: work-related asthma, isocyanates, occupational, inspections, medical surveillance

Introduction

Since the introduction of isocyanates in the 1930s, their application has increased worldwide. Workers are exposed to isocyanates in many industries, including: automotive and other plastic and foam-based parts manufacturing; construction; foundries; paint-using industries such as automotive repair shops; varnish-using industries such as furniture manufacturing; and in the manufacture of isocyanates themselves. The relationship between isocyanates and adverse health effects among workers exposed to them has been recognized in the scientific literature since the early 1950s. The spectrum of health effects from exposure to isocyanates ranges from dermatitis and allergic rhinitis to hypersensitivity pneumonitis, asthma, and, even death. Especially since the early 1980s, researchers have studied isocyanate-induced asthma from many perspectives including clinical, epidemiological, socioeconomic and industrial hygiene.

Several key points have been repeatedly documented: individuals may develop asthma from exposure to low levels of isocyanates; peak exposures such as spills or leaks can be responsible for acute onset of asthma either through sensitization or Reactive Airways Dysfunction Syndrome (RADS); monomers as well as prepolymers can cause work-related asthma; many sensitized workers remain working in isocyanates for financial reasons rather than take a cut in pay at a non-exposure job; and, perhaps most importantly from a clinical perspective, the sooner an individual is recognized as having isocyanate-induced asthma and removed permanently from such exposures the greater the likelihood that the asthma symptoms will improve or cease [1-10]. In an effort to address some of the documented health effects of the isocyanates, new forms have been developed, such as naphthalene diisocyanate (NDI). However, the effect that these new forms of isocyanates will have on worker health has yet to be fully studied [11].

As the use of isocyanates, both the monomers and prepolymers, has increased over the last few decades, an increasing number of workers are potentially exposed to some type of isocyanate. The highest estimated number of workers exposed to isocyanates in the United States comes from a NIOSH Hazard Alert, and indicates at least 280,000 workers potentially exposed to isocyanates [12]. An estimated 5-10% of isocyanate-using workers will develop asthma [12]. Researchers are documenting that isocyanate-induced asthma is one of the main causes of occupational asthma worldwide [13-16].

In Michigan, isocyanates account for approximately 20% of the total cases of work-related asthma (WRA) reported to the state's occupational disease registry. Michigan has required the reporting of all known or suspected occupational diseases since 1978. In 1988, the state of Michigan received federal funding to conduct active surveillance of occupational diseases, including work-related asthma. Since that time, surveillance of work-related asthma in the Michigan work force has found that isocyanates account for the greatest number of work-related asthma cases identified in Michigan.

In this paper we will review the epidemiology of isocyanate-induced asthma among the Michigan work force; summarize the results of related work place follow up inspections; and discuss the importance of medical surveillance in the early detection and removal of sensitized workers.

Methods

Subjects

Michigan law requires physicians, clinics, hospitals and employers to report work-related diseases to the state. All individuals reported with asthma or symptoms consistent with asthma were administered a standardized telephone questionnaire that documented each case's work and exposure history, breathing symptom history, cigarette smoking history, and medical care and breathing medication history. The questionnaire also asked workers if they had been exposed to spills and leaks of isocyanates in their work area. A definition for what constituted a spill or leak, such as the amount, was not given to the worker. The questionnaire was developed specifically for this project and has been used since 1988.

Based on review by a board certified occupational medicine physician (KR) of the medical records and the telephone-administered questionnaires for the 1765 cases reported to the state with asthma or symptoms consistent with asthma from 1988-1998, 1336 (76%) were confirmed as having WRA per criteria developed by the National Institute for Occupational Safety and Health (NIOSH) [17]. Medical records typically consisted of breathing tests and recent progress notes from outpatient care or a discharge diagnosis from a hospitalization. This paper will examine the characteristics of 261 of those cases whose asthma was caused by isocyanates.

Work-Related Asthma Case Definition

The work-related asthma case definition was developed in conjunction with the National Institute for Occupational Safety and Health (NIOSH) and several states conducting work-related asthma surveillance [*17*]. The definition of work-related asthma was: (1) a diagnosis of asthma; and (2) an association between symptoms and work. The case definition allowed for four types of work-related asthma: work-aggravated asthma, reactive airways dysfunction syndrome (RADS), and occupational asthma with or without exposure to a known allergen. There are over 350 known WRA allergens that have been cited in the scientific literature [*18*].

Work Place Inspections

As part of Michigan's surveillance system for WRA, Michigan Occupational Safety and Health Act (OSHA) enforcement inspections were routinely conducted at facilities where individuals developed their asthma. Inspections were completed if: the facility was in Michigan and within Michigan OSHA jurisdiction; exposures were ongoing; if the index case's work-related asthma was not work-aggravated asthma (i.e., the case had to develop their asthma after beginning to work at the facility); and a similar inspection had not recently been conducted. The enforcement inspections typically conducted air monitoring for the suspected allergen, assessed compliance with state laws, and conducted a breathing symptom survey of the co-workers in similar exposures as the index case. After an inspection was completed, a copy of the Michigan OSHA inspector's findings was given to the facility that was inspected, to the union or worker representative for health and safety if no union existed, and to the physician who originally reported the index case.

Co-workers of the index cases from the WRA registry were interviewed during these inspections to assess the extent of breathing problems among similarly exposed individuals. At the 36 inspections where co-workers were interviewed, 730 co-workers completed a standardized questionnaire. All co-workers in the same area of exposure as the index case who were working at the time of the inspection were given the opportunity to complete the questionnaire.

The standardized questionnaire for co-workers was developed in 1988 and since then has been administered in 389 facilities to 7337 co-workers. The questionnaire asked questions regarding work history, medical care for respiratory problems, allergy history, cigarette smoking history and frequency of respiratory symptoms. The criteria for a worker to be classified as having breathing problems based on these co-worker interviews was the indication of being bothered at work by daily or weekly chest tightness, shortness of breath or wheezing, or if the worker indicated the development of asthma since beginning to work at the facility. Interviews were not performed at six of the 42 companies inspected because the staff person that performed these interviews was not available to accompany the Michigan OSHA enforcement inspector.

Air Sampling for Isocyanates

The Michigan OSHA permissible exposure limits for isocyanates vary by type of isocyanate. For the more frequently encountered isocyanates used in Michigan industry, methylene bisphenyl diisocyanate (MDI) has a ceiling limit of 0.02 parts per million (ppm); toluene diisocyanate (TDI) has an 8-hour time-weighted average (TWA) limit of 0.005 ppm and a short-term exposure limit (STEL) of 0.02 ppm; and hexamethylene diisocyanate (HDI) does not have a limit, although NIOSH and the American Conference of Governmental Industrial Hygienists (ACGIH) have a recommended TWA limit of 0.005 ppm. There are other isocyanate types that are regulated by Michigan OSHA. However, the only isocyanates types used at the 42 companies inspected were TDI, MDI and HDI.

In October of 1993, the Michigan OSHA program changed their sampling methodology for isocyanates by switching their sampling from a closed face with a 37mm glass fiber filter with a nitro reagent followed by HPLC/UV, based upon NIOSH method 347 to a three-piece open-faced cassette based upon OSHA methods 42 and 47. Prior to October of 1993, Michigan OSHA inspectors were not consistently using open-faced sampling, which may have resulted in the isocyanates contacting the cassette before they reached the filter and derivatizing agent (nitro reagent); this would have resulted in sampling results that were lower than the actual exposures.

Since that time 42 Michigan OSHA enforcement inspections were conducted from October 1993 through 1999, based on the 261 isocyanate-induced asthma cases identified through the WRA registry. A total of 160 breathing zone and ten area air samples for isocyanates were collected at 41 of the companies, compliance with Michigan OSHA laws was assessed at all 42 companies and confidential co-worker interviews were administered at 36 of the companies. The location and number of air samples that were collected was determined by the Michigan OSHA inspector who was assigned to that inspection. The intent of the Michigan OSHA inspector was to determine compliance with the OSHA permissible exposure limit (PEL) among co-workers in the area in which the index case worked.

Statistics

Mantel-Haenszel odds ratios were calculated to compare the risk of having symptomatic co-workers in companies with spills versus companies without spills. The Chi Square statistic was calculated to determine if there were any differences in the percentage of companies with symptomatic co-workers by isocyanate type.

Results

Case History

A 30-year-old female began working in the late 1980s at a company that made doors for houses and garages. She was exposed to MDI in her job, which was to sandwich the two sides of a door together and fill it with urethane insulation before taking them to a press. She was classified as a "urethane assembler." She wore rubber gloves and a paper filter mask, as well as safety glasses and safety shoes at work. She noted that the paper mask "didn't seem to work." She developed wheezing, chest tightness and shortness of breath approximately 2¾ years after beginning to work at the facility. Her symptoms were worse at work. She had no past history of asthma. An occupational medicine physician diagnosed her with occupational asthma. She went on medical leave 10 months after her symptoms first began. Approximately one year after she was last exposed to MDI her breathing symptoms were still present, although the symptoms were less severe. In addition, she was still taking asthma medications, but less frequently. She had smoked cigarettes for less than a year when she was 17 years old.

A Michigan OSHA enforcement inspection was conducted at her workplace. The plant had been in operation for 20 years. The company did not conduct any medical monitoring, including a questionnaire for respiratory symptoms, breathing tests or blood tests, of employees for sensitization to MDI. Five breathing zone air samples and two area samples for MDI were collected during the inspection; none of the samples had any MDI detected. The limit of detection for these samples ranged from 0.001 ppm to 0.005 ppm. During the inspection, 25 co-workers similarly exposed as the index case completed a breathing symptom questionnaire. Six of those individuals had daily or weekly chest tightness, shortness of breath or wheezing in relation to work. A medical monitoring program for workers exposed to MDI was recommended, and the six symptomatic co-workers were sent letters to their homes advising them to see their physician about their breathing symptoms. The company was cited for several violations of Michigan OSHA regulations including: the lack of a hazardous waste operations and emergency response plan; an incomplete blood borne pathogens exposure control plan; an incomplete hazard communication plan; and the lack of suitable eye wash and first aid facilities.

Interviews with 261 Isocyanate-Induced Asthma Cases

From 1988-1998, physicians, hospitals, workers' compensation or co-workers reported a total of 1765 individuals with known or suspected work-related asthma to the State of Michigan. Of the 1765 individuals identified, 1336 were confirmed as having work-related asthma. Approximately 20% (261/1336) of those individuals with WRA developed their asthma from exposure to isocyanates at work. Of the 261 isocyanate-induced asthma cases, 248 (95%) were classified as occupational asthma; 7 (3%) were classified as aggravated asthma; and 6 (2%) were classified as RADS. Over half (56%) of the 261 isocyanate-induced asthma cases were men and 79% were white. Sixteen percent of the 261 cases were African American; the remaining 5% were Asian, American Indian, or listed as "Other".

Approximately one third of the isocyanate WRA cases were from exposure to toluene diisocyanate (TDI). Table 1 shows the type of isocyanate exposure of the 261 cases.

Table 1. *Type of Isocyanate Exposure Among 261 Individuals Reported to Michigan, from 1988-1998*

Type of Isocyanate*	Number of Cases (Percent)	
TDI	84	(32)
MDI	69	(26)
HDI	14	(5)
TDI and MDI	10	(4)
NDI	8	(3)
Unknown Type	76	(29)
Total	261	

*TDI=toluene diisocyanate; MDI=methylene bisphenyl diisocyanate; HDI=hexamethylene diisocyanate; NDI=naphthalene diisocyanate.

Michigan has a large manufacturing sector, with 961000 workers, of which 272000 people were working in automotive manufacturing in 1999 [*19*]. The total working population in Michigan in 1999 was 4894000 individuals. The majority of the 261 cases were exposed to isocyanates at facilities involved in manufacturing, especially in automotive parts manufacturing. Over half (133/243) of the cases who worked at manufacturing facilities were reported by the medical departments at those facilities. Table 2 shows the types of industries where the isocyanate-induced asthma cases worked.

We examined the type of industry where exposure occurred by type of isocyanate used. The automotive manufacturing industry accounted for the highest percentage of cases exposed to TDI (73%, n=61/84), followed by the rubber and plastics manufacturing industry (12%, n=10/84). Automotive manufacturing also accounted for the greatest percentage of MDI-exposed individuals, with 52% (n=36/69), followed by foundries, with 17% (n=12/69). The automotive repair industry accounted for 14% (n=2/14) of the HDI-exposed workers; the automotive manufacturing industry accounted for 71% (n=10/14) of those HDI-exposed cases.

One hundred twenty-one (50%) of the 241 individuals with isocyanate-induced asthma where the use of health care services was known had presented at a hospital emergency room (ER) since their asthma symptoms began, with an average number of 4.9 ER visits. For 20 of the 261 individuals, the use of health care services was unknown. Sixty (25%) of the 241 individuals with known health care service use had been hospitalized at least once for their asthma symptoms, with an average of 2.8 hospital stays. We also examined the frequency of ER visits and hospital stays by the type of isocyanate to which the workers were exposed. Five of the eight (63%) NDI-exposed workers had at least one ER visit, and 39 of the 69 (57%) MDI-exposed workers, 40 of the 84 (48%) TDI-exposed workers, and 5 of the 14 (36%) HDI-exposed workers had at least one ER visit. Further, three of the eight (38%) NDI-exposed workers had at least one hospital stay, and 20 of the 84 (24%) TDI-exposed workers, 16 of the 69 (23%) MDI-exposed workers, and 2 of the 14 (14%) HDI-exposed workers had at least one hospital stay. These figures underscore the serious nature of this disease, especially MDI, which is typically viewed as a "safer" isocyanate since it is less volatile than TDI.

Table 2. *Industry of Isocyanate-Induced Asthma Cases Reported to Michigan, From 1988-1998*

Industry	Number of Cases (Percent)	
Automotive Mfg.	165	(63)
Miscellaneous Mfg.	24	(9)
Rubber and Plastics Mfg.	23	(9)
Chemical Mfg.	16	(6)
Foundry	15	(6)
Trade	7	(3)
Automotive Repair and Sales	6	(2)
Construction	2	(1)
Research Lab	2	(1)
Trucking	1	(<1)
Total	261	

Fifty-five of the 261 workers (21%) who developed isocyanate-induced asthma were still exposed to isocyanates in their job at the time of their telephone-administered medical questionnaire. One hundred ninety-two (74%) workers were no longer exposed to isocyanates. For fourteen (5%) individuals exposure status was unknown. Of the 192 workers no longer exposed to isocyanates: 41% (n=67) of the individuals had been reassigned to a new job; 18% (n=29) were on medical leave or workers' compensation; 14% (n=23) had quit their job for health reasons, either on their own or upon the advice of their physician; 4% (n=6) were fired; 2% (n=2) had a substitute chemical or engineering change to reduce their exposures; and the remaining 35 workers were no longer exposed to isocyanates for other reasons.

Despite removal from exposure, 78% of workers continued to experience breathing symptoms, although 51% experienced symptoms less often since they were removed from exposure. Table 3 shows the exposure status of the 261 isocyanate-induced asthma cases and the persistence of their symptoms.

Of the 192 workers who were no longer exposed to isocyanates at the time of interview, 68% were still using asthma medications to control their symptoms. Table 4 shows the exposure status and asthma medication use of the 261 isocyanate-induced asthma cases. Twenty-eight percent of the workers no longer exposed were using fewer asthma medications than when they were working with isocyanates.

Table 3. *Persistence of Symptoms of Isocyanate-Induced Asthma Cases Reported to Michigan, from 1988-1998*

	Total	Persistence of Asthma Symptoms	
		Yes	Less
Exposure Status*	#	# (%)	# (%)
Still Exposed	55	55 (100)	18 (33)
No Longer Exposed	192	149 (78)	97 (51)

*Information unknown for 14 cases.

Table 4. *Use of Asthma Medications of Isocyanate-Induced Asthma Cases Reported to Michigan, from 1988-1998*

	Total	Use of Asthma Medications	
		Yes	Less
Exposure Status*	#	# (%)	# (%)
Still Exposed	55	40 (73)	9 (16)
No Longer Exposed	192	130 (68)	53 (28)

*Information unknown for 14 cases.

Tables 3 and 4 illustrate the chronic nature of this condition and highlight the importance of secondary prevention. We also looked at the length of time it took from when an individual's breathing problems began at the company, to the time that they were no longer exposed to isocyanates. Overall, workers left the exposure an average of 40.31 months after their symptoms first began. By type of isocyanate to which a worker was exposed, the amount of time from the development of breathing problems to last exposure to isocyanates varied. HDI-users left an average of 26.4 months after their symptoms began; NDI-users left an average of 29.14 months after their symptoms began; MDI-users left an average of 44.93 months after their symptoms began; and TDI-users left an average of 48.91 months after their symptoms began.

Inspections at 42 Facilities

Since October of 1993, when the Michigan OSHA program instituted a new sampling methodology for the isocyanates, 42 work place inspections were conducted in relation to the 261 index cases reported to the occupational disease registry. At 41 of these 42 inspections air monitoring was conducted for isocyanates. An isocyanate level of TDI at one of these facilities was 0.005 ppm (TWA). Isocyanates levels at the other 40 companies were below 0.005 ppm (TWA). Despite these low levels of isocyanates noted during monitoring, individuals continue to develop asthma.

Another measure to help document the extent of the problem during these inspections was the administration of breathing symptom questionnaires to similarly isocyanate-exposed co-workers of the index cases. At 36 of the 42 facilities inspected, co-workers were interviewed about the presence of breathing symptoms at work or physician-diagnosed asthma since beginning to work with isocyanates. A total of 730 interviews were conducted during these inspections, and 172 (24%) indicated being bothered at work by daily or weekly shortness of breath, chest tightness or wheezing, or as having been diagnosed with asthma since beginning to work at the facility. Ten of the 36 companies where co-workers were interviewed had no co-workers with daily or weekly breathing symptoms or asthma. Of the remaining 26 companies with at least one symptomatic co-worker, the average percent of symptomatic co-workers per company was 26% (SD 13%).

Since all but one of the companies had measured isocyanate levels below Michigan OSHA permissible exposure limits, we examined the relationship of spills or leaks at companies with symptomatic co-workers. In the interviews with the 261 index cases, the interviewer asked whether the worker had been exposed to any spills or leaks of isocyanates. Table 5 compares the number of companies with symptomatic co-workers for which the index case indicated at least one isocyanate spill to companies with symptomatic co-workers where the index case had not been exposed to a spill or leak. A greater percentage of companies had symptomatic co-workers where the index case had reported at least one isocyanate spill (85%) than companies at which the index case indicated there had been no spills (65%), although this was not statistically significant. Again, although not statistically significant, a company was almost three times more likely to have symptomatic co-workers if the index case indicated a spill had occurred. At those companies where the index case reported at least one spill, the average percent of symptomatic co-workers identified at a company was 23% compared to 16% at companies where the index case indicated there had not been any spills; this was also not statistically significant.

We also examined the spill status of the companies inspected by the type of isocyanate used. Workers from TDI-using companies reported a higher percentage of spills (45% of 11 companies) than workers from MDI- or HDI-using companies (with 37% of 19 companies and 33% of 9 companies, respectively). Spill status was unknown for 3 companies.

Since isocyanate properties such as volatility differ by type of isocyanate, we examined the relationship of symptomatic co-workers by the type of isocyanate used at the facilities inspected. Table 6 shows the numbers of symptomatic co-workers by type of isocyanate used. A greater percentage of companies using MDI had symptomatic co-workers than companies using TDI or HDI. Further, the average percent of symptomatic co-workers at companies using MDI was higher than that of companies using TDI or HDI. The average duration of years exposed to isocyanates, by type of isocyanate used was 7.5 years for the interviewed co-workers in MDI-using companies, 7.1 years for the interviewed co-workers in the TDI-using companies, and 11.0 years for the interviewed co-workers in the HDI-using companies. Further, the percentage of interviewed co-workers who never smoked cigarettes was 40.8% in the MDI-using companies, compared to 33.9% in the TDI-using companies and 54.1% in the HDI-using companies.

Table 5. *Inspections at 36 of 42 Companies with Co-Worker Breathing Symptom Interviews, by Isocyanate Spill Status*

	One or More Spills/Leaks	No Spills
Companies with Symptomatic Co-Workers	11/13 (85%)	15/23 (65%)
	Odds Ratio: 2.93 (95% CL* 0.43 – 34)	
Average % Symptomatic Co-Workers	23%, SD 13% range 0 - 46%	16%, SD 17% range 0 - 60%
	Odds Ratio: 1.42 (95% CL 0.99 – 2.03)	

*CL Confidence Limit

For three companies the status of a medical surveillance program was unknown. The Michigan OSHA inspectors were able to document that 28 of the 39 facilities inspected did not have a medical surveillance program to monitor workers for sensitization to isocyanates. The other 11 companies did have such a medical surveillance program.

Of the 36 companies inspected where medical surveillance status was known and co-workers were interviewed, 19 of 25 (76%) of the companies had no medical surveillance program and had symptomatic co-workers. Seven of 11 (64%) of the companies had a medical surveillance program and symptomatic co-workers. Although not statistically significant, a company was less likely to have co-workers with breathing symptoms if they had a medical surveillance program (odds ratio: 0.55, 95% CL .092 – 3.29).

Table 6. *Inspections at 36 of 42 Companies with Co-Worker Breathing Symptom Interviews, by Type of Isocyanate*

Isocyanate Type	Companies with Symptomatic Co-Workers	Average Percent Symptomatic Co-Workers
MDI	15/18 (83%)	23%, SD 16%, range 0 – 60%
TDI	6/9 (67%)	15%, SD 13%, range 0 – 38%
HDI	5/9 (56%)	14%, SD 16%, range 0 – 30%
	(Chi-Square = 2.49, p=0.29)	(Chi-Square = 9.92, p=0.007)

Discussion

The Michigan surveillance system for WRA identified 261 cases of isocyanate-induced asthma. Michigan data shows that workers who develop isocyanate-induced asthma generally have severe and persistent asthma. While the majority of workers cease their exposure, some workers continue to work with isocyanates. Real life practical issues such as paying bills may override equally important medical issues such as removal from exposure to prevent further progression of disease. Since a newer sampling methodology was adopted in October of 1993, 42 inspections at facilities where these individuals worked and were exposed to isocyanates were conducted. Seven hundred and thirty co-workers of those index cases completed breathing symptom questionnaires as part of the enforcement inspections.

The Michigan experience of isocyanate-using facilities is probably not different from other states or from other countries. Being in compliance with the Michigan OSHA PEL does not preclude the development of work-related asthma. The reliance on air sampling data alone might give companies a false sense of security. The current Michigan and Federal work place standards for isocyanates do not include a requirement for medical surveillance, wage-retention for sensitized individuals, training, or procedures for the clean up of spills.

The longer an individual continues to be exposed to isocyanates after a diagnosis of work-related asthma, the greater the likelihood that their symptoms will persist [20]. A medical surveillance program to monitor symptoms among isocyanate-exposed workers should, therefore, be an integral part of any isocyanate-using facility's health and safety plan. In Michigan, however, 72% of the 42 companies inspected where isocyanate-induced asthma cases worked had no medical surveillance program. Several groups have recommended removal from exposure of sensitized individuals in consensus statements [21-25]. Medical surveillance should not take the place of engineering controls and safe handling practices, but should be in addition to those features.

There are limitations to this study. First, it is not possible to determine if a spill or low-level exposure was responsible for the development of each individual's asthma. No definition for spill or leak was provided to the index cases during the administration of the questionnaire. This might lead to misclassification of workplaces if the index cases used different definitions of "spill" or "leak". Assuming the misclassification was not in any specific direction, the effect of the misclassification would be to decrease the likelihood of finding an association. Further, sampling for isocyanates during inspections may not reflect typical exposure levels experienced by the workers on a day-to-day basis, and therefore might over or under estimate the workers' true exposures. One can conclude, however, that the presence of allowable air levels during a typical Michigan OSHA inspection does not preclude the presence of symptomatic workers. In addition, it was not possible to determine whether other possible asthma sensitizers were present in the workplace, which could also contribute to index case and co-worker breathing symptoms and obscure the potential effects of isocyanates.

The diagnosis of work-related asthma among individuals reported to the Michigan surveillance system followed the standard of medical care in the United States. This means the diagnosis in 95% of the reported cases was dependent on the history of a temporal relationship between symptoms and work. Only 5% of the reports had objective pulmonary function tests performed in relationship to work. Medical literature indicates that clinical history is sensitive but not specific [26-27].

High percentages of co-workers of the index cases with work-related asthma had daily or weekly symptoms of shortness of breath, chest tightness or wheezing identified through interviews conducted with these co-workers during Michigan OSHA enforcement inspections. The number of co-workers with work-related breathing problems is likely to be an underestimate of the true number of symptomatic individuals, since the extremely symptomatic individuals would presumably leave the job in addition to the fact that we did not classify individuals with monthly or less frequent breathing problems at work as positive. The extent to which workers leave the environment because of breathing problems was not known; this would under estimate both the magnitude and severity of breathing symptoms. On the other hand, because the questionnaire is a screening tool, not all symptomatic co-workers will have asthma let alone isocyanate-related asthma.

Recent studies of isocyanate-exposed workers have shown mixed results concerning the occurrence of respiratory symptoms at low-level exposures. Studies of MDI-exposed workers from wood product manufacturing facilities in the United States showed increased respiratory symptoms among workers in higher potential exposure areas [28] and in jobs below the OSHA permissible exposure limit of 0.02 ppm [29]. The first study measured actual air levels of isocyanates. Another study where isocyanate levels were measured and found to be well below 0.005 ppm found reductions in pulmonary function of the workers exposed, although there was no increase in the proportion of workers who developed respiratory symptoms or asthma compared to workers not exposed to isocyanates at the plant [30]. Different levels of exposure, isocyanate types and definitions of positive responses on questionnaires will all contribute to the variations found in the results of these studies.

Isocyanates play a large role in the manufacture of polyurethane products and there are few, if any options for substitution of other chemicals in their place. As new prepolymers are developed, the challenge to companies that manufacture and use these chemicals will be to determine the best way to ensure the safety of individuals who handle them. One way to work toward this challenge would be through the manufacturers of these chemicals to develop and promote medical surveillance programs for their own employees as well as for the employees at the companies to which they sell their product. It cannot be assumed that the new polymers will be safer than the original isocyanates. Further, despite its decreased volatility, our data does not suggest that MDI is "safer" than TDI. Although our results were not statistically significant, we found that a greater percentage of the MDI-exposed cases with isocyanate-induced WRA (57%) had at least one ER visit compared to the TDI-exposed cases (48%), and a similar percentage of hospital stays (MDI 23%, TDI 24%). In addition, the higher percentages of symptomatic co-workers of these index cases who were identified during inspections at the MDI-using companies were not explained by the duration of years worked in isocyanates or by cigarette smoking. The challenge to scientists and regulators will be to develop methods to sample for the new forms of isocyanates and institute new and more comprehensive workplace exposure standards to reduce the burden of isocyanate-induced asthma.

Acknowledgments

This paper was funded in part by a grant from the National Institute for Occupational Safety and Health (NIOSH) under cooperative agreement #U60-CCU502998-13.

The authors wish to acknowledge the tremendous support of the Michigan OSHA administrative and industrial hygiene staff. They also wish to acknowledge the support and interview staff at Michigan State University who handle the occupational disease reports, conduct interviews, and obtain medical records. They are: Larry Ansari, Amy Krizek, Tracy Murphy, Amy Sims and Ruth VanderWaals.

References

[1]   Leroyer, C., Perfetti, L., Cartier, A., and Malo, J. L., "Can Reactive Airways Dysfunction Syndrome (RADS) Transform into Occupational Asthma Due to 'Sensitisation' to Isocyanates?" *Thorax*, Vol. 53, No. 2, 1998, pp. 152-153.

[2]   Woellner, R. C., Hall, S., Greaves, I., and Schoenwetter, W. F., "Epidemic of Asthma in a Wood Products Plant Using Methylene Diphenyl Diisocyanate," *American Journal of Industrial Medicine*, Vol. 31, 1997, pp. 56-63.

[3]   Paggiaro, P. L., Vagaggini, B., Bacci, L., Carrara, M., Di Franco, A., Giannini, D., Dente, F. L., and Giuntini, C., "Prognosis of Occupational Asthma," *European Respiratory Journal,* Vol. 7, 1994, pp. 761-767.

[4]   Palczynski, C., Jakubowski, J., and Gorski, P., "Reactive Airways Dysfunction Syndrome," *International Journal of Occupational Medicine and Environmental Health*, Vol. 7, No. 2, 1994, pp. 113-117.

[5]   Gannon, P. F. G., Weir, D. C., Robertson, A. S., and Burge, P. S., "Health, Employment, and Financial Outcomes in Workers with Occupational Asthma," *British Journal of Industrial Medicine*, Vol. 50, 1993, pp. 491-496.

[6]   Marabini, A., Dimich-Ward, S. Y. L., Kennedy, S. M., Waxler-Morrison, N., and Chan-Yeung, M., "Clinical and Socioeconomic Features of Subjects with Red Cedar Asthma," *Chest,* Vol. 104, 1993, pp. 821-824.

[7]   Pisati, G., Baruffini, A., and Zedda S., "Toluene Diisocyanate Induced Asthma: Outcome According to Persistence or Cessation of Exposure," *British Journal of Industrial Medicine,* Vol. 50, 1993, pp. 60-64.

[8]   Vandenplas, O., Cartier, A., Lesage, J., Cloutier, Y., Perreault, G., Grammer, L. C., Shaughnessy, M. A., and Malo, J. L., "Prepolymers of Hexamethylene Diisocyanate as a Case of Occupational Asthma," *Journal of Allergy and Clinical Immunology,* Vol. 91, 1993, pp. 850-861.

[9]   Saetta, M., Maestrelli, P., Di Steffano, A., De Marzo, N., Milani, G. F., Pivirotto, F., Mapp, C. E., and Fabbri, L. M., "Effect of Cessation of Exposure to Toluene Diisocyanate (TDI) on Bronchial Mucosa of Subjects with TDI-induced Asthma," *American Review of Respiratory Disease*, Vol. 145, 1992, pp. 169-174.

[10]   Fabbri, L. M., and Mapp, C., "Bronchial Hyperresponsiveness, Airway Inflammation and Occupational Asthma Induced by Toluene Diisocyanate,*"* *Clinical and Experimental Allergy*, Vol. 21, Supplement I, 1991, pp. 42-47.

[11]   Fuortes, L. J., Kiken, S., and Makowsky, M., "An Outbreak of Naphthalene Di-Isocyanate-Induced Asthma in a Plastics Factory,*"* *Archives of Environmental Health*, Vol. 50, No. 5, Sept.-Oct. 1995, pp. 337-340.

[12]   National Institute for Occupational Safety and Health, *Request for Assistance in Preventing Asthma and Death from Diisocyanate Exposure*, DHHS (NIOSH) Publication No. 96-111, Cincinnati, March 1996.

[13]   Meyer, J. D., Holt, D. L., Cherry, N. M., and McDonald, J. C., "SWORD '98: Surveillance of Work-Related and Occupational Respiratory Disease in the UK," Occupational *Medicine (London),* Vol. 49, No. 8, 1999, pp. 485-489.

[14]   Bernstein, J. A., "Overview of Diisocyanate Occupational Asthma," *Toxicology*, Vol. 111, 1996, pp. 181-189.

[15]   Gannon, P. F. G., and Burge, P. S., "The SHIELD Scheme in the West Midlands Region, United Kingdom," *British Journal of Industrial Medicine*, Vol. 50, 1993, pp. 791-796.

[16]   Lee, H. S., Phoon, W. H., Wang, Y. T., Poh, S. C., Cheong, T. H., Tap, J. C., Lee, F. Y., and Chee, C. B., "Occupational Asthma in Singapore. A Review Cases from 1983-1990," *Journal of Epidemiology and Community Health*, Vol. 47, 1991, pp. 459-463.

[17]   Jajosky, R. A., Harrison, R., Reinisch, F., Flattery, J., Chan, J., Tumpowsky, C., Davis, L., Reilly, M. J., Rosenman, K. D., Kalinowski, D., Stanbury, M., Schill, D. P., and Wood, J., "Surveillance of Work-Related Asthma in Selected U.S. States Using Surveillance Guidelines for State Health Departments—California, Massachusetts, Michigan and New Jersey, 1993-1995," *Morbidity and Mortality*

Weekly Report Centers for Disease Control and Prevention, Surveillance Summaries, Vol. 48, No. SS-3, 1999, pp. 1-20.

[18] Table of Agents and Substances Which Can Cause Asthma, URL: http://www.remcomp.com.fr/asmanet/asmapro/agents.htm, AsmaNet, Paris, France, March 20, 2001.

[19] Michigan Department of Career Development/Employment Service Agency, Labor Market Analysis Section, Detroit, MI, 15 Feb. 2000.

[20] Chan-Yeung, M., and Malo, J. L., "Occupational Asthma," *New England Journal of Medicine*, Vol. 333, 1995, pp. 107-112.

[21] Chan-Yeung, M., "ACCP Consensus Statement Assessment of Asthma in the Workplace," *Chest*, Vol. 108, 1995, pp. 1084-1117.

[22] American Thoracic Society AD HOC Committee on Impairment/Disability Evaluation in Subjects with Asthma, "Guidelines for the Evaluation of Impairment/Disability in Patients with Asthma," *American Review of Respiratory Disease*, Vol. 147, 1993, pp. 1056-1061.

[23] National Heart, Lung and Blood Institute, National Asthma Education Program Expert Panel Report, "Guidelines for the Diagnosis and Management of Asthma," *Journal of Allergy and Clinical Immunology*, Vol. 88, 1991, pp. 425-534.

[24] Workshop on Environmental and Occupational Asthma, *Chest*, Vol. 98, 1990, pp. 145S-252S.

[25] AD HOC Committee on Occupational Asthma of the Standards Committee, Canadian Thoracic Society. "Occupational Asthma: Recommendations in Diagnosis, Management and Assessment of Impairments," *Journal of the Canadian Medical Association*, Vol. 140, 1989, pp. 1029-1032.

[26] Kraw, M. and Tarlo, S. M., "Isocyanate Medical Surveillance: Respiratory Referrals from a Foam Manufacturing Plant Over a 5-Year Period," *American Journal of Industrial Medicine*, Vol. 35, No. 1, Jan. 1999, pp. 87-91.

[27] Malo, J. L., Ghezzo, H., L'Archeveque, J., Lagier, F., Perrin, B., and Cartier, A., "Is the Clinical History a Satisfactory Means of Diagnosing Occupational Asthma?" *American Review of Respiratory Disease*, Vol. 143, 1991, pp. 528-532.

[28] Petsonk, E. L., Wang, M. L., Lewis, D. M., Siegel, P. D., and Husberg, B. J., "Asthma-Like Symptoms in Wood Product Plant Workers Exposed to Methylene Diphenyl Diisocyanate," *Chest*, Vol. 118, No. 4, October 2000, pp. 1183-1193.

[29] Woellner, R. C., Hall, S., Greaves, I., and Schoenwetter, W. F., "Epidemic of Asthma in a Wood Products Plant Using Methylene Diphenyl Diisocyanate," *American Journal of Industrial Medicine*, Vol. 31, 1997, pp. 56-63

[30] Akbar-Khanzadeh, F. and Rivas, R. D., "Exposure to Isocyanates and Organic Solvents, and Pulmonary-Function Changes in Workers in a Polyurethane Molding Process," *Journal of Occupational and Environmental Medicine*, Vol. 38, No. 12, December 1996, pp. 1205-1212.

John J. McAlinden[1]

Isocyanate Exposures in the United Kingdom

Reference: McAlinden, J. J., **"Isocyanate Exposures in the United Kingdom,"** *Isocyanates: Sampling, Analysis, and Health Effects, ASTM STP 1408,* J. Lesage, I. D. DeGraff, and R. S. Danchik, Eds., American Society for Testing and Materials, West Conshohocken, PA, 2002.

Abstract: Isocyanates are asthmagens and most studies of occupational exposures to isocyanates have concentrated on inhalation of the vapor or aerosol. However, exposure may also occur through skin contact with the aerosol or during the handling of liquid isocyanates. Prolonged contact may lead to irritation or contact dermatitis.

Isocyanates are not produced in the United Kingdom (UK). UK industry, however, currently imports between 90000 and 100000 tonnes of isocyanate per year. Isocyanates are widely used in the UK for the manufacture of flexible and rigid foams, fibers, coatings such as paints and varnishes, and elastomers. The UK industry occupational population potentially exposed to isocyanates is about 25000 workers and the overall use of isocyanates by UK industry is increasing slowly.

Traditionally, the occupational group considered to be most at risk from isocyanate induced occupational asthma is spray painters in the motor vehicle repair industry. Because of this, HSE has undertaken campaigns, targeted specifically at the motor vehicle repair industry, to identify how, why and for how long workers are exposed to isocyanates. The findings are discussed in this paper.

The distribution of cases of occupational asthma throughout UK industry by occupation and agent as reported to two UK occupational health databases over the last ten years are also discussed in this paper. Findings are then compared against industry's own occupational health data and sector population breakdowns. Consideration is also given to whether an underlying UK trend of increasing non- occupational asthmas could also influence the reporting of work-related cases.

Keywords: isocyanates, occupational exposures, occupational health data, occupational asthma.

Introduction

Toluene diisocyanate (TDI), methylene bisphenyl isocyanate (MDI) and hexamethylene diisocyanate (HDI) account for more than 90% of the commercial use of diisocyanates in the UK. They are widely used in the manufacture of flexible and rigid foams, fibers, coatings such as paints and varnishes, and elastomers.

---

[1] Health and Safety Executive, Stanley Precinct, Bootle, Merseyside L20 3QZ, UK.

Diisocyanates are increasingly used in the motor vehicle manufacture (manufacture of interior fittings and trim) and body repair industries and in the production of building insulation materials. In this paper, diisocyanates, as a group, will be referred to as isocyanates.

Isocyanates are not produced in the UK. Currently, UK industry imports between 90000 and 100000 tonnes of isocyanate per year (Te/yr) for consumption by UK industry and the exposed occupational population is about 25000 workers.

Isocyanates are asthmagens and most studies of occupational exposures to isocyanates have concentrated on inhalation of the vapor or aerosol. However, exposure may also occur through skin contact during the handling of liquid isocyanates. Prolonged contact may lead to irritation or contact dermatitis.

Health Effects

The development of asthma symptoms after exposure to isocyanates does not usually take place right away. It generally happens after several months or years of breathing in the chemical. Once a person contracts the disease, however, their condition is irreversible and symptoms can occur either immediately after they are exposed to the chemical or several hours later. If the symptoms are delayed, they are often most severe in the evenings or during the night, so workers may not realise exposure to isocyanates is making them ill. Further exposures can lead to permanent lung damage. Subsequent attacks may also be triggered by non-workplace exposures to agents such as tobacco smoke or cold air. These attacks may continue even if exposure to isocyanates ceases.

UK Legislative Background

From 1969 to 1979, both TDI and MDI had ceiling limits of 0.02 ppm (0.14 mg/m^3) based on the American Conference of Governmental Industrial Hygienists (ACGIH) Threshold Limit Value (TLV). Subsequently, these recommended values were extended to all isocyanates. In 1984, the UK Health and Safety Executive (HSE) recommended a two part control limit of 0.02 mg/m^3, 8 hour time-weighted average (8 hr TWA) and 0.07 mg/m^3 (10 minute reference period) for exposure to free isocyanate groups. The two part control limit became a Maximum Exposure Limit (MEL) of 0.02 mg/m^3 (8 hour TWA) and Short Term Exposure Limit (STEL) of 0.07 mg/m^3 (10 minute reference period) on the introduction of the Control of Substances Hazardous to Health (COSHH) regulations in the UK in 1989 and in 1997 the 10 minute reference period for the STEL was extended to 15 minutes.

UK Enforcement Background

HSE provides guidance [1] on the precautions which need to be taken to prevent or adequately control exposures to isocyanates as required by COSHH. This guidance draws attention to the health hazards which could result from exposure to isocyanates and is particularly aimed at employers and managers of people potentially exposed to isocyanates in the course of their work.

During 1990, HSE carried out a survey to examine the effectiveness of control measures for isocyanates under COSHH. Eighty-five companies, representing a wide cross-section of isocyanate users, were inspected and all were aware of COSHH; 91%

were aware of the fact that a MEL existed for isocyanates and 62% knew the numerical value. Only 6% of the firms consulted had changed to isocyanate-free processes while 81% used respiratory protective equipment (RPE) for control of exposure. Engineering controls were used by 89% while 76% used both engineering controls and RPE. As a consequence of this initiative, 2% of the companies were prosecuted for failing to comply with COSHH and Improvement Notices were issued to 19% of the companies (Improvement and Prohibition Notices are legally enforceable and check visits are automatically made by HSE Inspectors to confirm compliance).

During 1996/97, HSE issued 41 Improvement or Prohibition Notices to companies for failing to comply with COSHH when working with isocyanates; 23 of the notices were issued to motor vehicle body repair shops. The other 18 notices were issued to a wide cross-section of other isocyanate users such as plastics moulding, metal coating or adhesives application.

During 1997/98, a further 69 notices were issued, 50 to motor vehicle body repair shops and 19 to other isocyanate users.

Over the two year period 1996/98, 92% of notices issued to motor vehicle body repair shops applied to activities involving the spraying of isocyanates whereas only 24% of notices issued to other isocyanate users applied to activities involving the spraying of isocyanates. The notices were issued to firms who failed to:

     v   provide health surveillance for employees working with isocyanates;
     v   prevent or control exposure of employees to isocyanates;
     v   make a suitable and sufficient assessment of risk for employees working with isocyanates.

During this period 1996/98, three successful prosecutions were taken by HSE Inspectors because of exposure to isocyanates; two prosecutions were for a failure to make a suitable and sufficient assessment of risk for employees working with isocyanates and one was for a failure to provide health surveillance.

UK Industry Isocyanate User Groups

Isocyanates Manufacturing Sector

There is no isocyanate production in the UK but at least 23 companies world-wide produce TDI and MDI. There has been a steady increase in use of isocyanates by UK industry over the last twenty years and this trend in growth (3% to 5% per annum) is set to continue.

Flexible Foam Manufacturing Sector

The flexible foam manufacturing industry is the biggest single user of TDI in the UK. About 17000 tonnes/yr of TDI are used to manufacture about 60000 tonnes/yr of flexible foam. Manufacture is centered at about six large block plants and the exposed occupational population is in the range of 200 to 300. Manufacture of the foam is undertaken remotely under controlled conditions. The TDI and other chemical components are accurately metered and fed individually to a mixing head which deposits the chemical mix onto a paper-lined conveyor. A foam is produced which then expands. As the foam expands, it sets into a continuous block which is carried away on the conveyor. The block formed on the conveyor moves along a curing tunnel which is under exhaust ventilation, the paper is stripped off and the continuous block is cut into standard lengths which are transferred to a curing warehouse. Once cured, the foam is cut up for use in such items as furniture, mattresses, bedding, soundproofing insulation and sponges.

Flexible foams are also used in the production of shaped articles such as car seats. The dispensing process is essentially the same as that used to produce foam block but the mixing head incorporates an "on-off" device which enables the correct amount of chemical mix to be dispensed into an individual mould which is then conveyed to a curing station under exhaust ventilation.

A longitudinal study [2] was carried out between 1981 and 1986 on 780 workers from twelve factories to look for cases of lung decrement. The study concluded that the lung decrement observed in the workers was typical of those of non-isocyanate longitudinal studies. The study was repeated between 1991 and 1996 on the remainder of the original cohort still employed in the industry. This group numbered in excess of 400 and the repeat study was unable to discover any cases of work-related asthma in the cohort.

Rigid Foam Manufacturing Sector

The UK rigid foam manufacturing industry uses about 20000 tonnes/yr of MDI to manufacture about 40000 tonnes/yr of rigid foam.

Rigid foams are produced by injecting an MDI-based polyurethane mix into a mould. The foam forms *in situ* and the air escaping from the breather hole generally contains some free isocyanate. The plant used to produce rigid foam can be either a permanently installed factory unit or a portable or mobile unit. It can consist of either one or two pressurized containers connected to a dispensing gun. The foam may be applied by injection or spray.

Manufacture is centered at about six large block plants under controlled conditions and the exposed occupational population is about 100. Cured rigid foam from factory produced slabstock can be supplied for cutting into appropriate forms to provide pipe insulation or cavity insulation.

Rigid foam is widely used as an insulating material by the construction industry in two types of laminated product. It is sprayed onto plywood to form insulating board for use in roof spaces, wall cavities and floors. It is also used in the manufacture of steel-faced building panels where it is sprayed on the outer surface to provide a weatherproof covering, the inner surface to provide a decorative finish and injected into the interspace to provide thermal insulation.

Rigid foam insulation is also used in the manufacture of smaller numbers of laminated units for the construction industry (items such as doors, for example) on a non-continuous production basis. There are about 200 smaller firms involved in such operations with an exposed population of about 1000. There are three major suppliers of copper hot water cylinders in the UK who spray rigid foam insulation onto their cylinders before despatch for sale. These companies employ an exposed population of about ten sprayers. The *in situ* application of sprayed rigid foam to both outer and inner roofing surfaces to provide weatherproofing and structural integrity is an area of significant growth. This work is carried out by about forty specialist contractors with an exposed occupational population of about 150 sprayers. Sprayers at such companies are provided with full face air-fed RPE and personal protective equipment (PPE) and are trained in the correct methods of working by the suppliers of the spray systems who provide training packages with their product systems. It is claimed by the rigid foam manufacturing sector that exposures in this area are controlled to as low a level as is reasonable and practicable. HSE has no exposure data in this area.

The provision of thermal insulation to combat global warming and the growing trends in renovation of older buildings lead the trade bodies to predict a sector growth of up to 10% for rigid foams. Other applications for rigid foam products include buoyancy aids, interior fixtures and trim for motor vehicles, and packaging.

Motor Vehicle Manufacturing and Repair Sector

The motor vehicle manufacturing sector uses isocyanates mainly in areas such as the production of interior fittings and trim and bonding of windscreens to their rubber sealant strip. This work is carried out by specialist subcontractors and not at the vehicle assembly plant.

There is some limited use, however, of paints containing isocyanates at vehicle assembly. This happens when, on final inspection, a finished vehicle's paintwork is found to be scratched and needs touching up. Paints containing isocyanate are used for this work as the finished repair can be heated locally to about 50°C using a portable infrared lamp. If paints that did not contain isocyanates were used (as in original manufacture) the vehicle would need to be returned to the production line to be stripped of all fixtures and fittings and be sent back through the oven-based paint curing process at about 150°C. Touch-up work is undertaken at a dedicated spray booth, provided with local exhaust ventilation (LEV), by a paint sprayer wearing full face air-fed RPE and PPE. One car manufacturer contacted had measured personal exposures of less than 0.001 mg/m^3 (8 hr TWA) at such operations. Industry claims that there is no evidence to link the vehicle manufacturer's paint sprayers with cases of asthma.

Most vehicle repair and body shops use urethane paints containing isocyanates because they produce a durable, hard and glossy finish and can be cured locally at low temperature without damaging the vehicle interior fittings. Isocyanates are typically found in the hardener of two-part paints and primers. Isocyanates are present in two forms, monomer and prepolymer. Frequently, the isocyanate monomer content is indicated in product data information, but this is only a small fraction of the total unreacted isocyanate present in hardeners. Both forms of unreacted isocyanate present a risk to health when they enter the breathing zone during paint spraying.

Industry contacts have estimated there could be about 10000 vehicle repair and body shops in the UK consuming approximately 1500 tonnes/yr of urethane paints containing isocyanates with an exposed occupational population of about 20000 paint sprayers. There are seven principal paint suppliers to the industry and the trends indicate a steady increase in use of isocyanates.

HSE guidance [*1*] to paint sprayers is to wear properly maintained full face air-fed RPE and PPE and to work inside a properly maintained spray booth. Traditionally it has been the case that smaller body shops, often unknown to HSE and operating on a low budget, fail to meet these requirements. Developing trends in the industry indicate a decrease in the number of vehicle body shops and numbers have fallen from about 15000 to 10000 over the last five to ten years. This decrease is due to the insurance companies deciding to direct insurance repair work to their own contracted body shops. This is leading to a gradual but inevitable "squeezing out of business" of the smaller operators. The larger franchised body shops and major independents tend to employ the industry trade associations' Health Surveillance program and argue that cases of sensitization are to be found in the smaller independent operators.

Printing and Lamination Sector

There are about 50 UK companies specializing in lamination work with an exposed population of about 200 workers. There is a wide range of applications for MDI from the production of flexible packaging for the food industry to circuit boards for the electronics industry and consumption is steady. There are pressures, however, on the industry to introduce TDI for food packaging as this would shorten the time taken for the packaging to cure. Also, the development of a flexible design of circuit board is underway now and this should stimulate a further increase in demand for isocyanates used to produce such boards. The work undertaken does not involve spraying and is carried out remotely under controlled conditions.

Exposure Data

During the period 1985 to 1996, HSE visited 50 places of work categorized as isocyanate users (note: no sampling visits were made in 1992) to carry out sampling and monitoring for isocyanates. The industries visited are summarized at Table 1.

Table 1 - *Breakdown by year and industry of HSE visits involving the sampling and monitoring of isocyanate*

	'85	'86	'87	'88	'89	'90	'91	'93	'94	'95	'96	Total
Motor vehicle body repairs	1	1	1		1		1		4			9
Application of adhesives	2			1		1	2			1		7
Laminates production	1		1							1		3
Flame bonding of materials	2											2
Clothing fabric manufacture		1										1
Rigid foam manufacture		1	2	1	1	1	2		1			9
Application of coatings to metalwork		1	1	1		3		1				7
Production of foundry moulds			1	1								2
Elastomer production			3	1	2				1		1	8
Road surfacing (construction)						1	1					
Total	6	4	9	5	4	6	6	1	6	1	2	50

The mean 8 hr TWA exposures measured by HSE at the 50 workplaces visited are listed at Table 2. No trends in exposures can be identified from this data.

Table 2 - *Mean 8 hr TWA exposures measured at workplaces*
(bld - below limit of detection)

Year	Mean 8 hr TWA (mg/m^3)	Number of samples taken	Range (mg/m^3)
1985	0.005	20	bld to 0.035
1986	0.0003	4	bld to 0.001
1987	0.003	34	bld to 0.02
1988	0.007	24	bld to 0.03
1989	0.001	10	bld to 0.03
1990	0.037	37	bld to 0.37
1991	0.009	31	bld to 0.211
1992	no data	-	-
1993	0.03	2	0.01 to 0.05
1994	0.029	11	bld to 0.17
1995	0.0084	2	0.0037 to 0.013
1996	bld	4	-

Human Health Data

SWORD Data

The Surveillance of Work-related and Occupational Respiratory Disease (SWORD) reporting system was introduced in the UK in 1988. SWORD data is collected from over 1000 participating chest physicians of whom 65 members form a "core" group who report monthly; the remainder are allocated at random to report in only one of 12 monthly samples. Occupational respiratory disease data provided from SWORD is therefore subject to sampling error.

There were 410 isocyanate asthma cases recorded on SWORD in the last three available reported years, 1995-1997, compared with 413 in the period 1992-1994. SWORD data for isocyanate asthma cases therefore provides no evidence for a falling off in numbers of such cases.

For the two-year period, 1997-1998, there were 234 cases reported although 1998 data is not fully complete. For this, most recent, two-year period, the number of isocyanate-related asthma cases, with the industry sector, are shown in Table 3.

Table 3 - *Cases of isocyanate induced asthma reported to SWORD in 1997/98 by industry sector*

Industry sector	Cases of asthma
Manufacturing (includes wood products, paper products, rubber, plastics)	71
Motor vehicle manufacture	24
Publishing, printing and reproduction of recorded media	13
Sale, maintenance and repair of motor vehicles, retail sale of fuel	41
Public administration and defense; compulsory social security	39
Miscellaneous	27
Unknown	19
Total	234

DSS Data

Work-related asthma caused by exposure to isocyanates was prescribed as an industrial disease under the Department of Social Security (DSS) Industrial Injuries Scheme in March 1982. The number of new cases of work-related asthma caused by exposure to isocyanates, as reported to the DSS Industrial Injuries Scheme, since then are listed at Table 4.

Table 4 - *Incidence of work related asthma caused by isocyanate exposure, as reported to the DSS Industrial Injuries Scheme, before and after the introduction of COSHH*

Year	Number of new cases before COSHH	Year	Number of new cases after COSHH
1982	45	1989	72
1983	74	1990	73
1984	51	1991	95
1985	46	1992	121
1986	48	1993	108
1987	60	1994	121
1988	64	1995	98
		1996	83

The figures for incidence of work related asthma caused by exposure to isocyanates prior to the introduction of COSHH in 1989 seem to show fluctuations around a fairly steady level. In the first years after isocyanate-induced asthma was prescribed as an industrial disease they were probably affected by the spread of knowledge about the availability of compensation which makes interpretation of the figures more difficult.

The figures for incidence of work-related asthma caused by exposure to isocyanates after the introduction of COSHH do not show any evidence for a fall. The figures for the period 1991-1996 are consistent with minor year-to-year fluctuations around an underlying steady rate.

A breakdown by industry of cases of DSS-prescribed occupational asthma where the named agent is isocyanates has been provided and is reproduced at Table 5. It covers the years 1995 and 1996 and lists all industries where four or more cases occurred.

Table 5 - *Breakdown by industry of cases of DSS prescribed occupational asthma where the named agent is isocyanates for the years 1995 and 1996*

Industry	1995	1996
Manufacture of motor vehicles	15	9
Repair of motor vehicles	13	16
Manufacture of chemical products	10	2
Manufacture of pumps and compressors	6	2
Other services	6	4
Construction	6	9
Manufacture of fabricated metal products	5	4
Manufacture of rubber and plastics	4	6
Electricity, gas, steam and hot water supply	2	5
Other	31	26
Total	98	83

It is probable that the figures for the two years reported for Repair of motor vehicles (29), Manufacture of pumps and compressors (8) and Manufacture of fabricated metal products (9) are for workers employed to spray isocyanate paints onto metal surfaces. From talking to industry contacts, we believe that the figures reported for Manufacture of motor vehicles (24), Manufacture of rubber and plastics (10) and Construction (15) are for workers employed to spray isocyanates into moulds to form rigid foams. These two types of work involving spraying isocyanates could, therefore, account for half the reported cases.

Discussion

Only a small number of sampling and monitoring visits have been made by HSE. These visits were not randomly selected but measured data from these visits provides no evidence of a reduction in workplace exposures since the MEL was introduced.

Data available from both SWORD and the DSS give no indication of any decrease in occupational asthma. Reporting levels may be higher now than before COSHH because the introduction of COSHH increased levels of awareness of work related asthma. There is also an underlying trend to an increase in non-occupational asthmas and this increase may have influenced the reporting of work-related cases.

The motor vehicle repair (MVR) sector is of the opinion that problems with isocyanate exposure lie with failures to control exposure of paint sprayers. They also believe that use of isocyanate paints is set to increase for the foreseeable future. HSE considers that existing guidance [1] on control of exposures for isocyanates sprayers is adequate and, if followed, would allow industry to comply with the MEL. Other industry groups do not believe that they have an occupational asthma problem and the longitudinal study [2] supports this claim for the flexible foam industry.

Analysis of the reported data indicates that there is an incidence of occupational asthma amongst paint sprayers of about 1:1000 per annum, but they appear not to be the group most at risk. The claims by some other industry sectors that they do not have problems of occupational asthma is at odds with the data from SWORD and the DSS presented in Tables 3 and 5.

Both the SWORD and DSS data show that MVR asthmas account for just under 20% of all isocyanate-induced asthmas. About 20000 workers are exposed to isocyanates in motor vehicle repair (predominantly sprayers) and about 5000 workers are occupationally exposed in the foam manufacture and use industries, motor vehicle manufacture, printing and laminating industries. If this number is doubled to take into account workers exposed in other smaller industry sectors not contacted, this gives a total of 10000 workers exposed outside the motor vehicle repair sector. These 10000 workers give rise to the remaining 80% of isocyanate induced asthmas and indicate an incidence of about 1:100 per annum. Within this overall grouping, there are likely to be pockets of higher incidence of asthma. Lamination may be a problem area, but the different ways the information has been classified makes direct comparison difficult.

Analysis of the summarized data suggests a high incidence of asthma cases in areas other than the MVR industry: and similar results are obtained from analysis of both the SWORD and DSS data. This is not the view put forward by the five major industry sectors contacted, however.

Conclusions

Measured data from HSE visits provide no evidence of a reduction in workplace exposures to isocyanate. The number of occupational asthma cases from isocyanate use shows no signs of a reduction.

Analysis of the summarized health data shows that incidence of asthma is not restricted to the motor vehicle repair industry, and may, in fact, be greater for other groups. This conclusion is contrary to the view given by several industry sectors.

A strategy for a survey of all UK companies who distribute or use isocyanates has therefore been developed jointly by HSE and appropriate UK industry and trade union bodies. The survey will investigate and clarify how isocyanates are handled through the supply chain, the measures taken to control exposure and the effectiveness of these measures. It will also provide an estimate of ill health associated with different uses.

References

[1]   Health and Safety Executive, "Isocyanates: Health Hazards and Precautionary Measures," Guidance Note EH16, HSE Books, Sudbury, Suffolk, UK, ISBN 0-7176-1184-1.

[2]   Clark, R. L., Bugler, J., McDermott, M., Hill, I. D., Allport, D. C., and Chamberlain, J. D., "An Epidemiology Study of Lung Function Changes of Toluene Diisocyanate Foam Workers in the United Kingdom," *International Archives of Environmental Health, 1998, 71: 169-179.*

Anne Harman Chappelle,[1] Ronald N. Shiotsuka,[2] and Michael J. Bartels[3]

Some Limitations in the Use of Urine Biomonitoring for Measuring TDI Exposure

---

Reference: Chappelle, A. H., Shiotsuka, R. N., and Bartels M. J. **"Some Limitations in the Use of Urine Biomonitoring for Measuring TDI Exposure,"** *Isocyanates: Sampling, Analysis, and Health Effects, ASTM STP 1408*, J. Lesage, I. D. DeGraff and R. S. Danchik, Eds., American Society for Testing and Materials, West Conshohocken, PA, 2002.

Abstract: Although reliable methods are available to monitor the concentrations of TDI in workplace air, some investigators use urine testing methods to determine if a worker has been recently exposed to TDI. This method relies on sophisticated analytical techniques in which various metabolic or breakdown products of TDI present in urine are converted in the laboratory to a derivative, toluene diamine (TDA). The total amount of converted TDA measured in the urine has been proposed as an estimate of exposure to TDI, assuming that an individual has not been exposed to another source of TDA.

Results of TDI biomonitoring may be difficult to interpret and the following points must be considered: 1) The pathway for TDI elimination has not been fully investigated in humans, a direct correlation between TDI air monitoring and urine TDA levels is not feasible; 2) Studies of TDI exposures in the workplace have not consistently shown a good correlation between air exposure levels and biomonitoring results; 3) Biomonitoring for TDI exposure by measuring converted TDA in urine does not identify peak exposures which may be more relevant to pulmonary sensitization; 4) Urine monitoring results for TDI exposure have not been correlated to adverse health effects and no biological monitoring limit has been established for TDI; 5) The detection of converted TDA in laboratory assays on processed urine samples does not necessarily reflect the presence of free TDA in the body, therefore it may unintentionally introduce concerns related to airborne TDI exposures.

Data generated from urine biomonitoring for exposure toTDI must be interpreted with caution and significant questions remain regarding the relevance of these studies for quantitative TDI exposure assessment.

Keywords: TDI, urine biomonitoring, TDA

---

[1]Associate Toxicologist, Huntsman Polyurethanes, 286 Mantua Grove Road, West Deptford, NJ 08066 Email: anne_h_chappelle@huntsman.com.

[2] Principle Research Scientist, Bayer Corporation, 17745 South Metcalf, Stillwell, KS 66085.

[3]Technical Leader- Analytical Chemistry, Toxicology & Environmental Research and Consulting, The Dow Chemical Company, 1803 Building, Midland, Michigan 48674.

Introduction

Toluene diisocyanate (TDI) is a chemical compound that reacts rapidly with polyols in the presence of amines to produce flexible polyurethane foam. TDI has been well studied [1, 2] and appropriate safety precautions and engineering controls are available to protect workers and the public (www.isofacts.org, www.polyurethane.org). Potential worker exposure to TDI is usually evaluated by ambient air monitoring. Occasionally, biological monitoring has been used. The American Conference of Governmental Industrial Hygienists (ACGIH) has established threshold limit values (TLVs) for worker exposure to TDI in workplace air [3] on the basis of protection from the development of sensitization. Biological exposure limits, such as German Biologischer Arbeitsstoff-Toleranz-Wert (BAT) values or ACGIH Biological Exposure Indicators (ACGIH BEIs) have not been established for TDI, which suggests that urine biomonitoring has not been accepted as a reliable tool for quantitating exposure.

Some epidemiology data provide evidence that prolonged exposure to TDI at levels above exposure guidelines may result in decreased lung function [4, 5]. Persons exposed to episodic high levels of TDI may become sensitized and may experience adverse pulmonary effects on re-exposure to TDI at levels below the exposure limit [6]. To prevent the loss of lung function and induction of sensitization in workers potentially exposed to TDI, ACGIH has established TLVs of 36 $\mu g/m^3$ (time weighted average) and 140 $\mu g/m^3$ (short-term exposure limit) [3] based on the work of Diem [4]. In a recent study by Ott [7], the TDI unit and referent employees were nested within a larger cohort of 2133 site employees previously studied for mortality and their respiratory health was examined. In agreement with other studies [5, 8-10] conducted in workplaces with exposures ranging up to the TLV TWA and where active medical surveillance and exposure monitoring programs were in place, there was little evidence of a relation between exposure to TDI and either forced vital capacity (FVC) or forced expiratory volume in the first second (FEV$_1$) decrement.

Three large studies of cancer incidence or mortality have been conducted in the polyurethane foam industry [11-14]. These studies do not show a consistent relationship between cancer incidence and diisocyanate exposure [15]. Although an oral gavage study concluded that, under the conditions of the study, TDI in corn oil was carcinogenic in rats [16], long term inhalation studies in rats and mice showed no evidence of carcinogenicity following exposure up to 1.068 mg/m^3 for 2 years [17]. The different outcomes result in a range of classifications for International Agency for Research on Cancer (IARC), National Institute for Occupational Safety and Health (NIOSH) and the ACGIH. IARC has classified TDI as 2B (carcinogenic in animals) [18, 19], while NIOSH, based on the gavage studies has classified TDI as a carcinogen [20], and finally ACGIH as A4 [1], not classifiable as a human carcinogen. Humans exposed to much lower concentrations of TDI in workplace air are unlikely to experience any significant carcinogenic risk.

A number of air monitoring methods have been developed to determine ambient concentrations of TDI in workplace air [21-23]. With appropriate expertise and equipment, the measurement of airborne levels of TDI can be reliably performed [24].

Rosenberg and Savolainen first described and investigated biomonitoring of TDI-exposed workers in 1985 [25]. Since then, biological monitoring for TDI has been sporadically used to address workplace scenarios where individuals are involved in different processes with large variation of exposure levels. Historically, urine sampling has been done at single time points or at collection intervals up to 28 hours post exposure. Sophisticated analytical and modeling methods are then used to estimate the total amount of the chemical that might have been inhaled or absorbed during a work shift. The advantage of this approach is that, in principle, the "total dose" for an individual may be estimated.

Biomonitoring for toluene diamine (TDA) in the urine of exposed workers suggests that the metabolic pathway for TDI elimination has been fully characterized to establish a quantitative relationship between TDI and TDA. The metabolism of TDI has not been thoroughly investigated in humans. Theoretically, due to the highly reactive nature of TDI, *in vivo* it is likely that it will react with the tissue it initially reaches rather than being distributed throughout the body unchanged. This is supported by inhalation studies using ^{14}C TDI in guinea pigs, showing that radioactivity in the blood is associated with a plasma component of 71 kDa [26, 27]. Although biochemical studies indicate that the hydrolysis of TDI to TDA can occur, it is a minor metabolic pathway because of competing reactions of TDI primarily with -NH, -SH and -OH groups of organic molecules in the respiratory tract and blood [28]. The most rapid reaction is with amines to form ureas, which results in minimal biological consequence due to their non-reactive nature, but still contribute to the total TDA extracted from urine. Furthermore, any TDA that is formed may react with free TDI to form polyureas. Biochemical studies with radiolabeled TDI vapor by Kennedy [27, 29] and Timchalk [30] have demonstrated little or no free TDA. Measurement of hydrolyzed TDA could imply wrongly, that a considerable amount of a carcinogenic compound was generated in the body of these individuals and is now detected in urine. Doe and Hoffmann [31] presented a careful evaluation of the available data and the possible risk of cancer (*via* TDA) from TDI exposure. It is demonstrated that there is not an unacceptable risk of carcinogenicity in the workplace at the current TLV for TDI, which is further supported by data from three epidemiology studies [11-14].

Urine biomonitoring is a powerful tool, but must be taken into context of the technical limitations of the assay. The goal of an effective monitoring program is to reduce the occurrence of adverse health effects, and the usefulness of urine biomonitoring for TDA for the protection of human health from TDI over-exposure has not yet been fully demonstrated.

Measurement of TDA in Hydrolyzed Urine

There are several papers that describe methods for the analysis of various aromatic amines in biological matrices (i.e.: urine, blood, and plasma). These amines are known metabolites of various isocyanates. Analysis of these amines in representative biofluids may provide at least qualitative information on workers' exposure to the parent isocyanates.

Since it is well known that most of the aromatic amines in blood and urine exist as one or more conjugates, nearly all of the methods [*32-38*] require an initial chemical hydrolysis to cleave the conjugated product back to the free amine compound. The methods described by Brorson, Lind, Persson, and Skarping utilize an "overnight" (16-hour) acid hydrolysis in 3.6 N HCl at 100 °C. The method described by Maitre (1993) involves a 2-hour hydrolysis in 9.6 N HCl at 100 °C. Tinnerberg et al. (1997) utilized a 16-hour hydrolysis at 100°C in 1.7 M sulfuric acid whereas Lewalter and Biedermann (1994) utilized a 2-hour hydrolysis at 80 °C in 20% sulfuric acid. Griffin et al. [*39*] utilized a basic hydrolysis in 20% NaOH at 80 °C for 2 hours. However, only one of these groups has evaluated the efficiency of this hydrolysis step. Skarping et al. (1994) examined the effect of pH, acid strength, hydrolysis time and temperature on the efficiency of toluene diamine (TDA) liberation from the urine and plasma of TDI exposed workers. These authors report no degradation of 2,4- or 2,6-TDA isomers with their "standard" 16-hour hydrolysis in 3.6 N HCl. However, they do mention that they were not able to completely cleave all acid-labile precursors of TDA, even after 240 hours of hydrolysis. This group also compared acidic vs. basic hydrolysis, at 100 °C and 110 °C (16 hour), and found approximately 2-fold greater liberation of TDA under basic conditions than with the analogous acid hydrolyses. No data were presented on the completeness of basic hydrolysis. Even with the enhanced liberation of both 2,4- and 2,6-TDA following basic hydrolysis or extended (>24 hour) acidic hydrolysis, the majority of the published methods utilize a 2-16 hour acidic hydrolysis. As a result, all of the methods described in the references may afford incomplete hydrolysis of the analyte(s), resulting in an underestimation of the isocyanate metabolites in urine or blood.

The analytes were quantitated primarily as perfluro-acyl derivatives via gas chromatography, with either electron-capture [*40*] or mass spectral [*32-38*] detection. One method employed high pressure liquid chromatography analysis of underivatized TDA via electrochemical detection (HPLC-ECD) [*39*]. Mass spectral analysis afforded the most selective and sensitive detection for the TDA analytes, with detection limits of 0.05-0.1 ng/ml sample. The GC-ECD method afforded detection limits of 1 ng/ml urine or plasma for the 2,4- and 2,6-isomers of TDA. HPLC-ECD analysis of TDA afforded detection limits of 0.5 ng/ml urine for both TDA isomers.

Biomonitoring of Urine

TDI Exposures in a Laboratory Setting

Two publications describe investigations addressing the kinetics of TDA concentrations in urine after controlled inhalation exposures of human volunteers to TDI in a test chamber. The chamber air concentration was monitored by a paper tape monitor and supplemented by analytical determinations using wet chemistry methods. Furthermore, volunteers in both studies [*32, 36*] were exposed only to TDI vapor and not an aerosol containing TDI. The Skarping study (1991) investigated the feasibility of using hydrolyzed urinary TDA concentrations as a biomonitor of TDI exposures in humans. Five male subjects who had no symptoms of urinary infection, respiratory disease, or history of atopy, and had normal renal clearance were exposed to a vaporized mixture of 2,4-TDI (48%) and 2,6-TDI (52%) in a test chamber for 7.5 hours. The mean air concentration was approximately 40 $\mu g/m^3$ (range of mean for individual subjects was 36 to 43 $\mu g/m^3$) and the estimated mean inhaled dose was 120 μg TDI. No amine (TDA) was found in the chamber atmosphere (<0.5 $\mu g/m^3$). Urine samples were stated to be stable for 6 months when acidified and stored at 4 °C (no data provided). The maximal elimination rate in urine occurred in the sample collected during the 6 to 8 hour span of a 7.5-hour exposure; the mean for 2,4-TDA was 0.6 μg/hour and that for 2,6-TDA was 1.0 μg/hour. The average urinary concentration for this same sampling period was 5.0 μg/l for 2,4-TDA and 8.6 μg/l for 2,6-TDA (no reference to measurement of urine creatinine was provided by the author). Only trace amounts of hydrolyzed TDA were detectable 24 hours after the start of exposure. The hydrolyzed urine samples revealed a biphasic pattern of TDA excretion. Half-life of the two phases was calculated using a semi-logarithmic plot of concentration vs. time (no further details were provided). The half-life for the initial phase had a mean of 1.9 hours for 2,4-TDA and 1.6 hours for 2,6-TDA. The half-life of the second phase was approximately 5 hours for both isomers. The cumulative amount of hydrolyzed TDA excreted in urine over 28 hours was estimated to range from 8 to 18% of the estimated dose. No hydrolyzed TDA was detected in pre-exposure urine samples.

A subsequent investigation by Brorson et al. [32] extended these findings to include investigation of hydrolyzed TDA elimination kinetics after exposure of subjects to different air concentrations of TDI. Two male subjects were exposed (4 hours/week) under controlled conditions to increasing mean air concentrations of 25, 50 and 70 μg TDI/m^3. Health evaluation revealed no symptoms of urinary infection or respiratory disease. Neither subject had a history of atopy or skin sensitization to TDI or prepolymers of TDI. No TDA formed by the potential hydrolysis of TDI was found in the chamber air. The chamber air contained a mixture of 30% 2,4-TDI and 70% 2,6-TDI. No TDA was found in pre-exposure urine samples. Urinary concentrations were given as mmol TDA/mol creatinine and excretion rate as μg/hour. Maximal elimination rates occurred at the end of the 4-hour exposure period with only trace amounts found after 24 hours. The 24-hour cumulative excretion of TDI ranged from 15% to 23% of the estimated inhaled dose. A biphasic elimination pattern was observed with the initial phase having a half-life of 5 hours for 2,4-TDA and 2.5 h for 2,6-TDA. The cumulative 24-hour urinary excretion showed a better relationship to air concentrations of TDI than did the rate of urinary excretion measured during the last 2 hours of exposure. A linear relationship was found between air concentrations of TDI and the 24-hour cumulative excretion of hydrolyzable TDA. Two sampling strategies are suggested by the investigators based on the observed relationship between air concentration and urinary TDA excretion rates of hydrolyzed TDA. The first is to obtain urine samples soon after end of exposure. Alternatively, 24-hour sampling of urine initiated at the start of each work-shift is considered by the investigators as the more reliable estimate of short-term exposures. Thus, the authors conclude biomonitoring of urinary hydrolyzable TDA only serves as an indicator of recent exposures to TDI because of the relatively rapid decline in measurable urinary TDA [32].

TDI Exposures in an Occupational Setting

A number of other investigators extended biomonitoring by sampling workers exposed to TDI during the course of a normal work-shift. Maitre et al. [*34*] studied nine workers exposed to an 80:20 (2,4-TDI: 2,6-TDI) mixture of TDI during foam production. The 8-hour mean air concentration of total TDI ranged from 9.5 to 94 $\mu g/m^3$. TDA concentration in urine was expressed as $\mu g/g$ creatinine. A linear relationship between air concentration of TDI and hydrolyzable TDA excreted in urine (urine sample collected at end of 8-hour shift) was found after log transformation of all data. The observation of a greater percent 2,6-TDA (relative to 2,4-TDA) in urine compared to percent of 2,6-TDI (relative to 2,4-TDI) in the exposure atmosphere for some subjects was suggested by the authors as reflecting contribution from dermal exposure. In another study [*35*], Persson et al. monitored 9 subjects at a flexible polyurethane foam manufacturing facility using 80:20 TDI. None of these subjects showed any pulmonary function decrement after exposure or have any TDI related health effects. The mean air concentration of TDI was generally between 0.4 and 4 $\mu g/m^3$ but values as high as 2000 $\mu g/m^3$ were also noted. The investigators were unable to relate the pattern of an individual subject's hydrolyzable TDA in urine with TDI exposures because of the limited number of air samples. The large inter-individual variability in hydrolyzed TDA elimination rates will limit the use of this data in back calculating the original exposure. Four workers had total hydrolyzed TDA elimination rates of 0.02 - 0.07 $\mu g/hour$ and two had an average of 0.1 - 0.3 $\mu g/hour$.

More recently, Lind et al. (1996) studied 4 workers involved in flexible foam production to examine the urinary elimination kinetics following exposure to 2,4-TDI and 2,6-TDI [*33*]. All subjects had normal spirometry values and none had dermal sensitization to TDI. Urine samples were collected before and after a 12-day holiday. The air concentration of TDI ranged from 10 to 120 $\mu g/m^3$. Plotting the natural log of concentration against time, the slope of a linear function fitted to the data was calculated. The time of urine sampling was not stated other than all urine was collected for the previous 24 hours. The half-life of hydrolyzed TDA in urine was 5.8 - 11 days for 2,4-TDA and 6.4 - 9.3 days for 2,6-TDA. Urinary levels of TDA are related to TDI exposure during the previous few hours [*32, 35, 36*], thus this study only provided information on a second elimination phase, which is likely related to the formation of adducts during metabolism.

Tinnerberg et al. studied 5 individuals at a flexible foam producing plant [*38*]. Air concentrations were continuously measured with a filter-tape instrument. The average air concentration was 29.8 $\mu g/m^3$ (12.5 - 79.9 $\mu g/m^3$). The authors report exposure of workers to both vapor phase TDI and to TDI associated with particles. Urine concentrations of hydrolyzed TDA were expressed as ug TDA/mmol creatinine. The urinary elimination pattern of hydrolyzed TDA was similar to those reported by other investigators but no statistical characterization was conducted. The authors conclude that air concentrations of TDI were not correlated to hydrolyzed TDA concentrations in urine [*38*].

Summary

The analytical procedures used by different investigators have several features in common. In each instance, the urine sample was hydrolyzed prior to chemical analysis for TDA. Samples stored at refrigerator temperature (4 °C) were acidified prior to storage. In one investigation, it was not stated that urine samples were acidified prior to storage but samples were kept at freezer temperatures (-20 °C) until analysis [*38*]. The biomonitoring methods described are sufficient for obtaining qualitative data on the relationship between isocyanate exposure and aniline-containing metabolites present in biofluids. The sample preparation and analysis techniques utilized provide acceptable selectivity and sensitivity for the analysis at the stated detection limits. However, since it has been reported that the hydrolysis of the TDA conjugates is probably incomplete [*37*], and further work is required to improve this step of the methods. Validation of hydrolysis efficiency should be performed with representative metabolites of TDI (*i.e.,* protein conjugate) and TDA *(i.e.,* diacetyl-TDA). An example validation experiment for hydrolysis efficiency has been performed with conjugates of the related aromatic amine, 4,4'-methylenedianiline (MDA), in human urine [*41*]. In the absence of hydrolysis efficiency data for the TDA isomers, the chemical analyses for TDA invariably resulted in measurements of only some of the hydrolyzable urinary TDA. Accordingly, no data on relative amounts of free TDA, conjugated TDA, metabolized TDI conjugates or currently unknown TDI-conjugates can be measured. Information on the non-hydrolyzable components would be potentially useful to explain the interindividual variability due to metabolic differences.

Noting the analytical limitations stated above, approximately 8 to 23% of the estimated inhaled dose of TDI appear to be excreted in urine over a 24-hour period. However, the incomplete hydrolysis of TDA conjugates suggests that these values may underestimate the actual percent excreted. In addition, the profiles of TDA elimination kinetics showed substantial inter-individual variability; thus, a 24-hour urine collection period was considered to yield a more accurate estimate of respiratory exposure to TDI than shorter sampling durations. The ideal sampling scenario is one which combines a longer total duration with multiple short sampling intervals to increase the accuracy of characterizing the elimination kinetics and possibly detecting peaks in exposure concentration. Generally, a biphasic pattern with a rapid initial elimination phase having a half-life of 1.9 to 5.0 hours for 2,4-TDA and 1.6 to 2.5 hours for 2,6-TDA was found. The slower elimination phase had a half-life of approximately 5 hours for both isomers. In one study where the hydrolyzed TDA elimination curve was apparently evaluated *in toto*, the half-life was reported to be 5.8 to 11 days for 2,4-TDA and 6.4 to 9.3 days for 2,6-TDA. It was not clear whether the longer half-life values were because of differences in statistical methods and sampling intervals/durations or sample hydrolysis procedures. Only trace amounts of hydrolyzed TDA was measurable in urine 24 hours after start of a 7.5-hour exposure. The elimination rate of hydrolyzed TDA in urine was thus dependent on exposure concentration and time of sampling relative to exposure.

In general, the sample size of many of these studies is small; relating air concentration of TDI to urine concentration of hydrolyzed TDA should be interpreted with caution. Using the TLV for TDI (36 μg/m^3) as an example, a corresponding value of 16.98 µg TDA/g creatinine in urine is predicted [*34*]. The differences seen in urinary levels are not necessarily due to peak exposure, but perhaps to inter-individual variation in metabolism, pharmacokinetics and a variety of life style factors (e.g. liquid intake, smoking) [*38*]. The controlled exposure studies were performed with TDI in the vapor phase, while real-world exposures may also be due to TDI associated with particles. Adequate information on the pharmacokinetics and metabolism of this compound by both of these exposure routes does not exist at this time. The usefulness of urine biomonitoring of TDA is further limited by the lack of adverse health effects correlated with the presence of hydrolyzable metabolites. The incomplete understanding of the metabolic pathway of TDI, and the paucity of data supports not establishing biological monitoring limits for TDI.

Conclusions

Biomonitoring assays have been developed and described to estimate TDI exposure by converting TDI and its urinary metabolites to TDA by vigorous acid or base hydrolysis, and measuring the amount of hydrolyzed TDA in the urine. However, the generated data must be interpreted with caution. Application of this methodology may only reflect average daily exposure while short-term peak exposures, which are considered critical with respect to occupational asthma, are less amenable to detection by these methods. The detection of TDA in urine samples after vigorous hydrolysis does not reflect the level of free TDA in the body; it estimates the combination of conjugated TDI derivatives, conjugated TDA and any free-TDA present in urine. Formation of TDA as a consequence of exposure to TDI at the TLV has not been shown to result in adverse health effects, including significant cancer risk. Correlation between air exposure levels and biomonitoring results in the workplace is not consistent and therefore would not assist in workplace monitoring that would result in the prevention of occupational asthma. The relevance of using urinary TDA measurements as a quantitative index for TDI exposure is questionable and further validation work is needed.

References

[*1*]   ACGIH, "Toluene Diisocyanate," in *ACGIH TLV Documentation*, 6th Edition, 2000, pp. 1581.

[2]   Karol, M. H., "Respiratory Effects of Inhaled Isocyanates," *Critical Reviews in Toxicology*, vol. 16, 1986, pp. 349-379.

[*3*]   ACGIH, "TLVs and BEIs: Threshold Limit Values for Chemical Substances and Physical Agents; Biological Exposure Indices,", 1999.

[*4*]   Diem, J. E., Jones, R. N., Hendrich, D. J., Glindmeyer, H. W., Dharmarajan, V., Butcher, B. T., Salvaggio, J. E., and Weill, H., "Five-Year Longitudinal Study of Workers Employed in a New Toluene Diisocyanate Manufacturing Plant," *American Reviews in Respiratory Disease*, vol. 126, 1982, pp. 420-28.

[5]   Jones, R. N., Rando, R. J., Glindmeyer, H. W., Foster, T. A., Hughes, J. M., O'Neil, C. E., and Weill, H., "Abnormal Lung Function in Polyurethane Foam Producers,

Weak Relationship to Toluene Diisocyanate Exposures," *American Reviews in Respiratory Disease*, vol. 146, 1992, pp. 871-77.

[6]   Malo, J. L., Ghezzo, H., and Elie, R., "Occupational Asthma Caused by Isocyanates: Patterns of Asthmatic Reactions to Increasing Day-to-Day Doses," *American Journal of Respiratory Care Medicine*, vol. 159, 1999, pp. 1879-83.

[7]   Ott, M. G., Klees, J. E., and Poche, S. L., "Respiratory Health Surveillance in a Toluene Diisocyanate Production Unit, 1967-97; Clinical Observations and Lung Function Analyses," *Occupational and Environmental Medicine*, vol. 57, 2000, pp. 43-52.

[8]   Weill, H., Butcher, B., and Dharmarajan, V., "Respiratory and Immunologic Evaluation of Isocyanate Exposure in a New Manufacturing Plant," Department of Health and Human Services, National Institute of Occupational Safety and Health (NIOSH), Cincinnati, OH 81-125, 1981.

[9]   Clark, R. L., Bugler, J., and McDermott, M., "An Epidemiology Study of Lung Function Changes of Toluene Diisocyanate Foam Workers in the United Kingdom," *International Archives of Occupational and Environmental Health*, vol. 71, 1998, pp. 169-70.

[10]   Musk, A. W., Peters, J. M., and Berstein, L., "Absence of Respiratory Effects in Subjects Exposed to Low Concentrations of TDI and MDI: A Reevaluation," *Journal of Occupational Medicine*, vol. 27, 1985, pp. 917-920.

[11]   Hagmar, L., Welinder, H., and Mikoczy, Z., "Cancer Incidence and Mortality in the Swedish Polyurethane Foam Manufacturing Industry," *British Journal of Industrial Medicine*, vol. 50, 1993, pp. 537-43.

[12]   Schnorr, T. M., Steenland, K., Egeland, G. M., Boeniger, M., and Egilman, D., "Mortality of Workers Exposed to Toluene Diisocyanate in the Polyurethane Foam Industry," *Occupational and Environmental Medicine*, vol. 53, 1996, pp. 703-07.

[13]   Hagmar, L., Stromberg, U., Welinder, H., and Mikoczy, Z., "Incidence of Cancer and Exposure to Toluene Diisocyanate and Methylene Diphenyldiisocyanate: A Cohort Based Case-Referent Study in the Polyurethane Foam Manufacturing Industry," *British Journal of Industrial Medicine*, vol. 53, 1993, pp. 1003-07.

[14]   Sorohan, T. and Pope, D., "Mortality and Cancer Morbidity of Production Workers in the United Kingdom Flexible Polyurethane Foam Industry," *British Journal of Industrial Medicine*, vol. 50, 1993, pp. 528-36.

[15]   Klees, J. E. and Ott, M. G., "Diisocyanates in Polyurethane Plastics Applications," *Occupational Medicine*, vol. 14, 1999, pp. 759-76.

[16]   National Toxicology Program, "Toxicology and Carcinogenesis Studies of Commercial Grade 2,4 (80%) and 2,6 (20%) - Toluene Diisocyanate," US Department of Health & Human Services, Research Triangle Park, NC 1986.

[17]   Loeser, E., "Long Term Toxicity and Carcinogenicity Studies with 2,4/2,6-Toluene-Diisocyanate (80/20) in Rats and Mice," *Toxicology Letters*, vol. 15, 1983, pp. 71-81.

[18]   International Agency for Research on Cancer, "IARC Monographs on the Evaluation of the Carcinogenic Risks of Chemicals to Humans," in *Some Chemicals Used in Plastics and Elastomers*, vol. 39. Lyon, France, 1986, pp. 287-323.

[19]   International Agency for Research on Cancer, "IARC Monographs on the Evaluation of the Carcinogenic Risks of Chemicals to Humans," in *Overall*

Evaluations of Carcinogenicity: An Updating of IARC Monographs Volumes 1 to 42, vol. Supplement 7. Lyon, France, 1987, pp. 72.

[20] National Institute for Occupational Safety and Health (NIOSH), *Toluene Diisocyanate (TDI) and Toluenediamine (TDA), Evidence of Carcinogenicity. Current Intelligence Bulletin 53*, vol. DHHS (NIOSH) Pub. No. 90-101; NTIS Pub.No. PB-90-192-915. Springfield, VA: National Technical Information Service, 1989.

[21] Mazur, G., Baur, X., Pfaller, A., and Rommelt, H., "Determination of Toluene Diisocyanate in Air by HPLC and Band-Tape Monitors," *International Archives of Occupational Environmental Health*, vol. 58, 1986, pp. 269-76.

[22] Rando, R. J., Hammad, Y. Y., and Chang, S. N., "A Diffusive Sampler for Personal Monitoring of Toluene Diisocyanate (TDI) Exposure; Part Ii: Laboratory and Field Evaluation of the Dosimeter," *American Industrial Hygiene Association Journal*, vol. 50, 1989, pp. 8-14.

[23] Lesage, J., Goyer, N., Desjardins, F., Vincent, J. Y., and Perrault, G., "Worker's Exposure to Isocyanates," *American Industrial Hygiene Association Journal*, vol. 53, 1992, pp. 146-53.

[24] Levine, S. P., Hillig, K. J. D., and Dharmarajan, V., "Critical Review of Methods of Sampling, Analysis and Monitoring for TDI and MDI," *American Industrial Hygiene Association Journal*, vol. 56, 1995, pp. 581-89.

[25] Rosenberg, C. and Savolainen, H., "Detection of Urinary Amine Metabolites in Toluene Diisocyanate Exposed Rats," *Journal of Chromatography*, vol. 323, 1985, pp. 429-33.

[26] Hill, B. L., Karol, M. H., and Brown, W. E., "The Fate of Inhaled [14c]-Toluene Diisocyanate in Sensitized Guinea Pigs," *Toxicologist*, vol. 6, 1986, pp. 15.

[27] Kennedy, A. L., Stock, M. L., Alaire, Y., and Brown, W. E., "Uptake and Distribution of 14c During and Following Inhalation Exposure to Radioactive Toluene Diisocyanate," *Toxicology and Applied Pharmacology*, vol. 100, 1989, pp. 280-292.

[28] Brown, W. E., "The Chemistry and Biochemistry of Isocyanates: An Overview," in *Current Topics in Pulmonary Pharmacology and Toxicology*, Hollinger, M. A., Ed. New York: Elsevier, 1987, pp. 200-225.

[29] Kennedy, A. L. and Brown, W. E., "Isocyanates and Lung Disease: Experimental Approaches to Molecular Mechanisms," *Occupational Medicine: State of the Art Review*, vol. 7, 1992, pp. 301-329.

[30] Timchalk, C., Smith, F. A., and Bartels, M. J., "Route-Dependent Comparative Metabolism of [14c] Toluene 2,4-Diisocyanate and [14c] Toluene 2,4-Diamine in Fischer 344 Rats," *Toxicology and Applied Pharmacology*, vol. 124, 1994, pp. 181-90.

[31] Doe, J. E. and Hoffmann, H. D., "Toluene Diisocyanate: An Assessment of Carcinogenic Risk Following Oral and Inhalation Exposure," *Toxicology and Industrial Health*, vol. 11, 1995, pp. 13-32.

[32] Brorson, T., Skarping, G., and Carsten, S., "Biological Monitoring of Isocyanates and Related Amines. IV. 2,4- and 2,6-Toluenediamine in Hydrolyzed Plasma and Urine after Test Chamber Exposure of Humans to 2,4- and 2,6-Toluene

Diisocyanate," *International Archives of Occupational and Environmental Health*, 1991, pp. 253-259.

[*33*] Lind, P., Dalene, M., Skarping, G., and Hagmar, L., "Toxicokinetics of 2,4- and 2,6-Toluenediamine in Hydrolyzed Urine and Plasma after Occupational Exposure to 2,4- and 2,6-Toluene Diisocyanate," *Occupational and Environmental Medicine*, vol. 53, 1996, pp. 94-99.

[*34*] Maitre, A., Berode, M., Perdrix, A., Romanazini, S., and Savolainen, H., "Biological Monitoring of Occupational Exposure to Toluene Diisocyanate," *International Archives of Occupational and Environmental Health*, vol. 65, 1993, pp. 97-100.

[*35*] Persson, P., Dalene, M., Skarping, G., Adamsson, M., and Hagmar, L., "Biological Monitoring of Occupational Exposure to Toluene Diisocyanate: Measurement of Toluenediamine in Hydrolysed Urine and Plasma by Gas Chromatography-Mass Spectrometry," *British Journal of Industrial Medicine*, vol. 50, 1993, pp. 1111-18.

[*36*] Skarping, G., Brorson, T., and Sango, C., "Biological Monitoring of Isocyanates and Related Amines. III. Test Chamber Exposure of Humans to Toluene Diisocyanate," *International Archives of Occupational and Environmental Health*, vol. 63, 1991, pp. 83-88.

[*37*] Skarping, G., Dalene, M., and Lind, P., "Determination of Toluenediamine Isomers by Capillary Gas Chromatography and Chemical Ionization Mass Spectrometry with Special Reference to the Biological Monitoring of 2,4-- and 2,6-Toluene Diisocyanate," *Journal of Chromatography*, vol. 663, 1994, pp. 199-210.

[*38*] Tinnerberg, H., Dalene, M., and Skarping, G., "Air and Biological Monitoring of Toluene Diisocyanate in a Flexible Foam Plant," *American Industrial Hygiene Association Journal*, vol. 58, 1997, pp. 229-235.

[*39*] Griffin, R. M., "Determination of Aromatic Amines in Urine by High Pressure Liquid Chromatography with Electrochemical Detection," *National Institute for Occupational Safety and Health*, Method L40067, 1997, pp.

[*40*] Lewalter, J. and Biedermann, P., *Aromatic Amines (Aniline, O-Toluidine, M-Toluidine, P-Toluidine, 4-Chloro-O-Toluidine, 2,4-Toluylenediamine, 2,6-Toluylenediamne, 4-Aminodiphenyl, 4,4"-Diaminodiphenylmethane)*, vol. 4: Verlagsgesellschaft mbH, Weinheim, FDR, 1994.

[*41*] Tiljander, A. and Skarping, G., "Determination of 4,4'-Methylenedianiline in Hydrolysed Human Urine Using Liquid Chromatography with Uv Detection and Peak Identification by Absorbance Ratio," *Journal of Chromatography*, vol. 511, 1997, pp. 185-194.

Athena T. Jolly,[1] Dieter Bramann,[2] and Hans-Peter Hoffarth[3]

Patch Testing for Isocyanates

Reference: Jolly, A.T., Bramann, D. and Hoffarth, H. P., "**Patch Testing for Isocyanates**," *Isocyanates: Sampling, Analysis, and Health Effects, ASTM STP 1408,* J. Lesage, I. D. DeGraff, and R. S. Danchik, Eds., American Society for Testing and Materials, West Conshohocken, PA, 2002.

Abstract: Dermatitis may occur as a result of exposure to chemicals in the workplace. Approximately 30 percent of cases of chemical dermatitis are classified as allergic contact dermatitis (ACD). Irritant contact dermatitis (ICD) is due to the irritant effect of chemicals and is much more common. Toluene diisocyanate (TDI) is one of many chemicals, which are both weak skin sensitizers and irritants. Diphenylmethane diisocyanate (MDI) has also been reported to be a skin sensitizer, but there is a question whether the skin reaction is due to a breakdown product, diaminodiphenylmethane (MDA), on the surface of the skin or to a cross reaction due to structural similarities. Biochemical data lends support to the latter rather than the former hypothesis. Patch testing is widely used to establish a causal relationship between ACD and a specific causative agent, and to differentiate between ACD and ICD, which often is not possible on clinical or even histological grounds. However, there are only a handful of chemicals available in standardized commercial trays in concentrations recommended by expert international organizations. Isocyanates are among the substances for which *no* generally accepted concentration has been adopted. Various concentrations have been recommended and are being used. As a consequence, there are real limitations in the interpretation of patch testing, particularly in the absence of expertise with the test methodology.

Keywords: allergic contact dermatitis (ACD); irritant contact dermatitis (ICD); patch testing; toluene diisocyanate (TDI); diphenylmethane diisocyanate (MDI); isocyanates; diisocyanates

---

[1]Consultant, Occupational and Environmental Health, 850 Penns Way, West Chester, PA 19382
[2]Medical Director, Occupational Health, Bayer AG, D-51368 Leverkusen, Germany.
[3] Occupational Health, Bayer AG, D-51368 Leverkusen, Germany.

Introduction

Dermatitis may occur as a result of exposure to chemicals in the workplace. Approximately 30 percent of cases of chemical dermatitis are classified as allergic contact dermatitis (ACD), caused by an immune response of the skin to the contact antigen[1, 2]. Irritant contact dermatitis (ICD), due to the irritant effect of chemicals, is much more common [1, 2]. Patch testing is widely used to establish a causal relationship between ACD and a specific causative agent, and to differentiate between ACD and ICD, which often is not possible on clinical or even histological grounds [3]. Toluene diisocyanate (TDI) and diphenylmethane diisocyanate (MDI) are two of the main diisocyanates. They are considered weak skin irritants[4]. It has been reported that relative few cases of ACD due to diisocyanates have been published in the scientific literature [4, 5]. This paper will be reviewing the majority of the papers on TDI and MDI contact dermatitis. In addition, we will focus on validation issues of patch testing for isocyanates. We will also be presenting the authors' experience with patch testing for isocyanates at the Bayer AG occupational medical department in Leverkusen, Germany.

Background

There currently are three widely used standardized patch tests: 1) Finn Chamber, 2) True Test, and 3) Epiquick. There is approximately 67 percent concordance of results among these methods [6]. In these tests, the suspected sensitizing agent is dissolved in a solvent and diluted to a concentration that will not cause irritation. A patch containing the diluted agent is applied to the skin and read at 48, 72 and 96 hours. The patch test is interpreted based on the observation of redness, itching and hardening of the skin at the site of the patch [6]. Given the importance of patch testing in diagnosing ACD, organizations, such as the International Contact Dermatitis Group, have recommended the use of a standard methodology for the test and its interpretation. However, standardized test concentrations have been proposed only for the most common of the approximately 100 environmental substances that are frequently associated with ACD. This is in contrast to the 2200 chemicals (out of 2-3 million chemicals) that have been identified as sensitizers [6].

Accuracy and Validity of Patch Testing

The accuracy or validity of the patch test is determined by its ability to truly diagnose those individuals with ACD, which defines the sensitivity of the test, and to eliminate those without it, which is the specificity of the test. A number of factors affect the

---

[4] Material Safety Data Sheets, available from TDI suppliers, provide additional health and safety information regarding this chemical.

accuracy of patch testing, including pre-selection of patients by a physician, selection of allergen, appliance vehicle, and, finally, proper technique [6]. Even when the test is performed using the recommended methodology and standardized panels of allergens on patients with high pre-test probability has ACD, false positive and false negative results may be encountered. There is greater uncertainty in interpreting patch test results when less common antigens are used, particularly if the test substance is also an irritant. The concentration that is used in the procedure is of great important for the following reasons[3]:

- At a given concentration of a material there might be 5 percent of individuals that will show a response but are still normal (false positives) and 5 percent of individuals with ACD to the material that will not respond (false negatives). This is considered to be good test performance.
- If an irritating concentration of the chemical is used in the testing, there will be an overlap of the irritant and the allergic responses. This overlap results in a much higher percentage of false positives, unless the concentration is set very low, which increases the risk of false negatives.

It is recommended that in order to establish the optimum concentration for any given allergen, 20 control subjects should be tested with several concentrations of the chemical [3]. This is not the case, even with the standard panels of allergens, where concentrations have been determined, mostly, empirically by dermatologists testing individuals with dermatitis and evaluating their response. The situation is worse with less commonly used allergens, where there is less experience with testing. Finally there may be a risk of sensitizing someone through patch testing, especially if it is not conducted using standard test panels. Accordingly, "such patch tests must not be applied indiscriminately since the induction of ACD may result in chronic disability for the test subject [3]."

Patch Testing for Isocyanates

Isocyanates are among the substances for which *no* uniformly accepted, standardized patch test concentrations have been adopted. Various concentrations have been recommended and used. For TDI concentrations have ranged from 0.1 to 2 percent [7, 8]. As examples of the difficulties of patch testing results, one case has been reported to have a negative result with TDI at 0.1 percent while at 0.5 percent concentration a positive result was seen [9]. At most, there has been only a handful of reports of ACD due to TDI, which has been characterized as a very weak skin irritant and sensitizer, causing dermatitis only as a consequence of grossly insufficient workplace hygiene [9]. In a series of 360 patients skin tested for ACD to plastics and glues, TDI was found to elicit an allergic response in 0.8% while inducing an irritant reaction in 1.9% of cases [10].

For MDI, concentrations have ranged among 0.01% [4], 1% [7] and 1.5-2% [10]. In several of the reports of ACD from MDI, the majority of individuals also reacted to MDA, the corresponding aromatic amine, which is known to be a skin sensitizer. The authors hypothesized that the primary sensitization in these cases could have been to

MDA, which might form as a result of hydrolysis of MDI on the skin [5, 8, 11, 12]. Alternately, the MDI reaction might reflect a cross-reaction due to structural similarities [5, 8, 12]. Biochemical *in vivo* data from skin exposure with ^{14}C MDI suggests that the formation of MDA from MDI on exposed skin practically does not occur [13]; therefore, cross reactivity to the patch testing antigens appears to be the more plausible explanation.

The largest series of patients reported were 360 patients patch tested for skin sensitization to 50 plastic and glue allergens in an occupational clinic in Finland between 1991-96. Only three of the patients (0.8%) reacted to MDI, ranking it a weak sensitizer when compared to more common allergens [10].

Patch Testing Reactions to Isocyanates in Leverkusen 1995-2000

The authors' experience with patch testing for diisocyanates has consisted of testing 16 individuals all employees of Bayer Ag. The tests were done with Finn Chambers on Scanpor placed on the patients' back, with one or two days' occlusion time. The following compounds were dissolved in petrolatum, MDI, TDI, Hydrogenated MDI (HMDI), Isophorone diisocyanate (IPDI). A commercial standardized panel was used for MDI and TDI with a concentration of 0.1%, according to the official recommendation of German Research Group. Preparations for HMDI and IPDI were made using concentrations of 0.1% and 0.01%. The results were read at 24, 48 and 72 hours. They were interpreted according to International Contact Dermatitis Research Group (ICDRG) recommendations. There were no positive responses to TDI and MDI. There was one positive response each to HPDI at 0.01% and IPDI at 0.1%. These results are consistent with the published literature in indicating that diisocyanates are weak sensitizers, with the exception of HPDI, which is described as a sensitizer in the MSDS based on animal data.

Conclusion

Patch testing can be used effectively as a diagnostic test if patients are properly selected and tested against standard series of allergens. Care in performing the test is important to reduce spurious irritant responses and requires experience with the test methodology. In the case of an irritant chemical, it is not always possible to differentiate between irritant and allergic contact dermatitis through patch testing. There are real limitations in the interpretation of the results when testing for substances such as isocyanates that do not have validated test concentrations. ACD from isocyanates is rather a rare condition and patch test results should always be correlated with the patient's symptoms and a dermatologist's examination. For MDI, care should be taken to avoid confounding of the test results by cross reactivity with the MDA antigen during patch testing.

References

[1]   ATSDR, *Skin Lesions and Environmental Exposures, Case Studies in Environmental Medicine 28*, 1993.

[2]   Nethercott, J. and Holness, L., "Occupational Allergic Contact Dermatitis," *Clinical Reviews in Allergy*, Vol. 7, 1989, pp. 399-415.

[3]   Nethercott, J., "Practical Problems in the Use of Patch Testing in the Evaluation of Patients with Contact Dermatitis," *Current Problems in Dermatology*, Vol. II, 1990, pp. 95-123.

[4]   Liden, C., "Allergic Contact Dermatitis from 4,4' Diisocyanatol-Diphenyl Methane (MDI) in a Molder," *Contact Dermatitis*, Vol. 6, 1980, pp. 301-302.

[5]   Alomar, A., "Contact Dermatitis from a Fashion Watch," *Contact Dermatitis*, Vol. 15, 1986, pp. 44-45.

[6]   Adams, R., "Patch Testing: Its Technique and Allergen Replacement" *Occupational Skin Diseases*, R. M. Adams, Ed., Second Edition, Philadelphia: Saunders, WB, 1989.

[7]   de Groot, A., "Patch Testing" *Test Concentrations and Vehicles for 3700 Chemicals*, Second Edition. New York: Elsevier, 1994.

[8]   Estlander, T., Keskinen, H., Jolanki, R., and Kanerva, L., "Occupational Dermatitis from Exposure to Polyurethane Chemicals," *Contact Dermatitis*, Vol. 27, 1992, pp. 161-165.

[9]   Diller, W., "Critical Review of the Human Toxicology of TDI," International Isocyanate Institute, Manchester, UK III Report 11198, 1998.

[10] Kanerva, L., Jolanki, R., Alanco, K., and Estlander, T., "Patch Test Reactions to Plastic and Glue Allergens," *Acta Derm Venerol*, Vol. 79, 1999, pp. 296-300.

[11] Tait, C. and Delaney, T., "Reactions Causing Reactions: Allergic Contact Dermatitis to an Isocyanate Metabolite but Not to the Parent Compound," *Australasian Journal of Dermatology*, Vol. 40, 1999, pp. 116-117.

[12] Rothe, A., "Contact Dermatitis from Diisocyanates," *Contact Dermatitis*, Vol. 26, 1992, pp. 285-286.

[13] Liebold, E., Hoffmann, H., and Hilderbrand, B., "MDI: Study of Absorption after Single Dermal and Intradermal Administration in Rats," International Isocyanate Institute, Manchester, UK, III 11341 126, 1999.

William E. Brown,[1] Shereen Gamaluddin,[2] and Amy L. Kennedy[3]

Antibody Testing: Analysis of the Specificity of Antibody Detection in a Non-Diisocyanate-Exposed Population

Reference: Brown, W. E., Gamaluddin, S., and Kennedy, A. L., **"Antibody Testing: Analysis of the Specificity of Antibody Detection in a Non-Diisocyanate-Exposed Population,"** *Isocyanates: Sampling, Analysis, and Health Effects, ASTM STP 1408,* J. Lesage, I. D. DeGraff, and R. S. Danchik, Eds., American Society for Testing and Materials, West Conshohocken, PA, 2002.

Abstract: The detection of specific antibodies (IgE and IgG) in the sera of some workers exposed to diisocyanates is not always consistent and often is not well correlated with a disease state. This is particularly a concern for the testing of TDI-exposed worker populations where the intensity of the specific antibody response is low. The present study was performed to examine the baseline antibody response in a population with no known exposure to TDI. Sera from 30, non-exposed individuals were screened for specific IgG and IgG4 antibodies using a variety of synthetic antigens. Specific and nonspecific inhibition of antigen binding was performed to determine the specificity of the antibody response. One of the serum samples showed a response greater than two standard deviations above the mean for each of the test antigens. All sera except the latter sample showed generalized antigen recognition that could not be specifically inhibited. These results suggest that within the general population, nonspecific reactions can compromise the specificity of diisocyanate antibody testing.

Keywords: diisocyanates, antibody response, antibody specificity, IgG, IgG4, TDI

[1]Professor, Department of Biological Sciences, Carnegie Mellon University, 4400 Fifth Avenue, Pittsburgh, PA 15213.

[2]Student, Department of Biological Sciences, Carnegie Mellon University, 4400 Fifth Avenue, Pittsburgh, PA 15213.

[3] Research Biologist, Department of Biological Sciences, Carnegie Mellon University, 4400 Fifth Avenue, Pittsburgh, PA 15213.

Introduction

The diagnosis of diisocyanate-induced occupational asthma has been difficult to achieve through traditional immunologic screening methods. In the case of the diisocyanates, antibody-screening methods such as ELISA or RAST have often given inconsistent results when correlated to clinical symptomology or specific inhalation challenge data [1-8]. The wide spectrum of associated respiratory diseases [9-13] and the differential reactivity of diisocyanates further complicates the issue [14]. Toluene diisocyanate (TDI)-exposed asthmatic workers, for example, have frequently been among the lowest responders in antibody screening studies [3, 4, 7, 8]. Many studies also analyze response groups by combining all data regardless of the specific diisocyanate involved and use limited numbers of individuals for control groups thus further complicating the literature.

Low numbers of positive antibody responders in TDI worker populations and inconsistent results between laboratories can be explained, only in part, by differences in conjugate preparation. Other confounding issues include the time of the collection of test sera, the treatment of test sera, and the methods used for antibody detection, characterization and response interpretation. Again, problems arise when individual laboratories differ in methodologies used. An initial study of specific antibody responses in TDI-exposed workers and a non-exposed population demonstrated variable antibody response levels in both study groups [15]. The high responses observed within the control population resulted in an elevated mean that complicated the classification of experimental samples into diagnostic groups. To improve the accuracy of the antibody measurements, it is therefore essential to evaluate the specific nature of the high responses in the control sera. The present study is an analysis of antibody screening for specific IgG and IgG4 antibodies using diisocyanate-HSA conjugates in a population of thirty individuals with no known exposure to diisocyanate compounds. Other test antigens such as a trimellitic anhydride-HSA conjugate, HSA and rye grass allergen were also included to evaluate generalized antibody recognition. Specific and nonspecific inhibition assays were performed to determine the specificity of any antigen recognition that was one standard deviation above the mean for the population. The results suggest that within the general population, nonspecific reactions can compromise the specificity of diisocyanate antibody testing and thereby impact the reliability of these methods for asthma diagnosis or determination of diisocyanate exposure.

Experimental Methods

Control Population Two independent sets of sera were used for this study. The first set was made up of 9 serum samples (ID #: 78, 80, 81, 88, 89, 96, 100, 102, 104) from individuals identified as non-exposed, non-asthmatics. These were provided by Dr. Jean-Luc Malo (Hopital Du Sacre'-Coeur De Montreal, Canada). The second set of

22 sera was purchased from Biological Specialty Corporation (BSC) (Colmar, PA). Sera in this group were from individuals with no known exposure to isocyanates. A donor questionnaire was completed for each donor and Table 1 is a compilation of information from the donor profiles supplied by the BSC.

Table 1 - *Summary of BSC Donor Profiles*

sera #	age	sex	occupation	smoker
171	24	F	housewife	*
172	41	M	blast operator	
173	21	M	forklift operator	*
174	35	M	laborer	*
175	26	F	phlebotomist	
176	27	F	customer service	
177	19	F	tellemarketer	
178	64	F	none	
179	21	M	landscaper	*
180	19	F	nursing assistant	
181	20	F	nurses aid	
182	29	F	tellemarketer	*
183	41	M	dishwasher	*
184	34	M	cashier	*
185	21	F	cashier	*
186	44	F	school bus driver	
187	35	F	housewife	*
188	41	F	bartender	*
189	24	F	lifeguard	
190	46	M	none	*
191	18	F	student	
192	22	F	clerk	

mean   30.545   males/smokers = 7/6
stdev   11.795   females/smokers = 15/5

Test Antigen Preparation

Preparation of TDI-HSA Conjugate 55 -The general protocol for the preparation of conjugate 55 (c55) is as follows. A stock TDI solution was made consisting of 2 ml of 2,4-TDI (Fluka Chemical Corp., Milwaukee, WI) in 5.8 ml of acetone and used immediately. Two ml of the stock TDI solution was added to a solution of 1 gram of

human serum albumin (HSA) (Sigma Chemical Company, St. Louis, MO) in 200 ml of
0.05M sodium borate buffer, pH 9.4, and the mixture was reacted for one hour with
stirring at room temperature. The reaction was quenched by addition of 200 ml of 2M
ammonium carbonate. The quenching reaction was allowed to proceed for 30 minutes
at room temperature. The final solution was dialyzed against four changes of distilled
H_2O. The conjugate in water was stored at $-20°C$.

Preparation of TDI-HSA Conjugate 56 - The general protocol for the preparation of
conjugate 56 (c56) is as follows. 0.05 grams of HSA were added to 10ml of 8% sodium
bicarbonate, pH 8.39. 41µl of pure TDI was added directly to the HSA solution and
the mixture was stirred at room temperature, in the hood, for one hour. The solution
was dialyzed four times against phosphate buffered saline (PBS), pH 7.2. The
conjugate in PBS was stored at $-20°C$.

Preparation of 4-4´ Methylene bis Phenylisocyanate (MDI)-HSA Conjugate 68 - The
synthesis of conjugate 68 (c68) followed that described for conjugate 56 with the
following exception. 84.5 µL of heated 4,4'-MDI monomer was used in place of the
TDI.

Preparation of Trimellytic Anhydride (TMA)-HSA Conjugate 100 (c100) - One gram
of HSA was added to 200 ml of 9% $NaHCO_3$ (chilled in ice water at 0° C). One gram
of TMA (Acros Organics, Geel, Belgium) was slowly added while stirring. The
reaction proceeded for 60 minutes at 0° C. The solution was dialyzed four times
against distilled water. The TMA conjugate in water was stored at $-20°C$.

Preparation of Rye Grass Allergen (c116) - 3 mg of Rye Grass from Allergon
(Angelholm, Sweden) was suspended in 1 ml PBS. The suspension was allowed to
settle for 20 minutes. The supernatant from this solution was used in the ELISA
assays. Comparisons were made between the supernatant and the suspended rye grass
solutions and their measurable protein concentrations were found to be equal. Both the
supernatant and suspension when used as antigens in the ELISA assay resulted in
equal responses to sera. In addition, SDS PAGE analysis of both samples yielded
equal patterns.

Test Antigen Characterization

Concentration Determination - Pierce MicroBCA and BCA Protein Assay Reagent
Kits (Pierce, Rockford, IL) were used to determine the protein concentration of the
conjugates. In addition to the BCA tests, a standard Lowry assay was performed on
each of the conjugates and the rye grass extracts. In all three assays, standard curves
were generated using HSA (Fraction V, Sigma Chemical Company, St. Louis, MO) as a
control.

SDS PAGE - Test antigens were analyzed on 10% polyacrylamide SDS gels [*16*].
Unmodified HSA and molecular weight marker proteins were used to characterize the
size distribution of the reaction products.

Isoelectric Focusing - Test antigens were also analyzed by isoelectric focusing using a pH 4-6 gradient [*16*]. HSA was run as a standard to measure differences in isoelectric point and homogeneity of the test antigens.

Immunologic Screening

Total IgG Concentration - The total IgG concentrations of all of the serum samples were determined using an immunodiffusion assay kit from The Binding Site (San Diego, CA). Sera were tested for specific IgG or specific IgG4 antibodies using enzyme-linked immunoabsorbent assay (ELISA) [*17*]. Anti-IgG (code AP004, lot 023067) and anti-IgG4 (code MP007, lot 6497) antibodies were obtained from The Binding Site. A titration assay of the secondary antibody was performed to ensure that the linear range of absorbance was being used.

ELISA Protocol - Test antigens (50 µg/well) were incubated in PBS in a 96 well plate (Greiner) overnight at 23° C. Wells were washed three times with PBS-Tween (0.1 ml Tween 20 in 200 ml PBS) and incubated one hour with either a milk blocking solution (MBS) (1% Non-Fat Dried Milk in PBS) or bovine serum albumin (BSA) blocking solution (1% in PBS) at room temperature. Except where noted, all ELISA were performed using MBS as the blocking agent. Wells were washed three times with PBS-Tween and then incubated for two hours with a sera/gelatin mixture at a 1:50 or 1:100 dilution of sera in PBS-(0.3%)gelatin. Wells were washed six times with PBS-Tween. Secondary antibody (anti-IgG or anti-IgG4) was added at a dilution of 1:3000 in PBS-Tween and incubated for one hour. Wells were washed 5 times with PBS-Tween. A substrate solution (30 mg 1,2-phenylene diamine (Aldrich Chemical Co., Milwaukee, WI), 50 ml citrate buffer, pH 5, 25µL 30% H_2O_2) was added and the reaction was quenched after 5 min. using 1M H_2SO_4. The plate was read with an automated microplate reader (Model Elx800, Bio-Tek Instruments, Winooski, VT) set at an absorbance of 490 nm. Each plate contained blank wells that were developed in parallel and then subtracted from each sample value for the plate.

Assay Linearity Assessment - Further characterization of the ELISA was performed to determine the linearity of the color development using phenylene diamine as substrate with hydrogen peroxide. A linear regression analyses of the rate of absorbance increase over the 5-minute incubation period with the substrate for different serum concentrations (range of serum dilutions: 1:50 to 1:800) indicates that the assay itself is linear (correlation coefficient range: 0.914 to 0.998) with time over the five-minute incubation period tested in this experiment. In addition, linear regression analysis of the relationship between the serum dilution and the slope of the absorbance response with time (slope of linear regression) shows excellent linear correlation (r^2=0.997). This indicates that there is a direct relationship between absorbance response and the amount of serum present even in the 1:50 dilution of serum.

Inhibition Assays - ELISA inhibition assays were also performed on select sera. The protocol for the assays was as described above. In these assays, c56 was bound to the plates during the overnight incubation. Three different concentrations of each inhibitor were mixed with sera prior to the sera incubation period. Inhibitors included TDI-HSA conjugates 55 (c55) and 56 (c56), TMA-HSA conjugate 100 (c100), MDI-HSA conjugate 68 (c68), and HSA. Serum 152 from an TDI-exposed, asthmatic individual was used as a positive control for the inhibition studies.

Calculations

Serum Response Standardization - Comparisons of serum responses to various conjugates with either anti-IgG or anti-IgG4 as a secondary antibody were made by performing assays in duplicate wells on duplicate plates. Sample distribution on plates was designed such that more than one common serum overlapped between plates. The average of sera absorbances for a specific conjugate was determined for each serum on each plate. For two plates that contained a large overlap, a ratio of the specific averages for a particular serum from one plate to the next was calculated. The average of all the calculated ratio values gave rise to a normalization factor by which the values of one plate were multiplied to standardize absorbance readings between two plates. All calculations were performed using Microsoft Excel 98.

Normalization Calculation - In order to correct for total IgG concentration of the sera, a normalization calculation was performed. The values for all absorbances for each serum and conjugate were divided by the total IgG concentration value that was experimentally found for the corresponding serum.

Results

Test Antigen Characterization - Preliminary characterization of the test antigens was performed to show similarities and differences in size and charge distribution between different antigens. Individual conjugate heterogeneity was also examined by these methods. SDS-PAGE was used to determine the molecular size variations between the different conjugates. The SDS-PAGE electropherogram showed that, with reference to unmodified-HSA, c55 has a characteristic lower apparent molecular weight due to intramolecular crosslinking. c56 demonstrates a smaller decrease in apparent molecular weight and appearance of heterogeneity with the presence of small amounts of dimer presumably resulting from intermolecular crosslinks. c100 has only the monomer molecule with an apparent increase in molecular weight relative to unmodified HSA. This is consistent with addition of molecular mass to HSA without intramolecular crosslinking since TMA is monofunctional.

Isoelectric focusing was used to measure the charge differences between the test antigens relative to unmodified HSA. With reference to unmodified HSA, c55 has the lowest isoelectric point consistent with modification of primary amines at pH 9.4.

c56 also has a lowered isoelectric point and its diffuse banding suggests a significantly greater heterogeneity relative to unmodified HSA. c100 has a single homogeneous species with a lowered isoelectric point relative to unmodified HSA again consistent with the monofunctional modification of specific amino groups by TMA.

Serum Sample IgG Response to Test Antigens - The serum samples were screened for their IgG response to a variety of test antigens including two different TDI-HSA conjugates (c55, c56), a TMA-HSA conjugate (c100), a MDI-HSA conjugate (c68), and an aqueous extract of ryegrass allergen (c116). Unmodified HSA was also tested. Figure 1 is a set of bar graph plots of representative IgG responses. Table 2 is a compilation of those sera that exhibit IgG responses either ≥ the mean plus the standard deviation (stdev) (+) for the individual test antigen or ≥ the mean plus twice the standard deviation (2stdev) (++) for the individual test antigen.

Table 2 - Compiled Responses ≥ (mean + stdev) (+)
and ≥ (mean + 2stdev) (++) within a Specific Group.

sera\	IgG						IgG4				
conjugate	c55	c56	c100	c68	c116	HSA	c55	c56	c100	c116	HSA
171	+	+	+	+	+	+	+	++	++	+	+
178	++	++	++	++	++	++	++	++	++	++	++
185				+							
186							+	+		++	
189				+	+						
190							+	+		+	+
96	+	+	+	+	+						
100			+		+						

Serum Sample IgG4 Response to Test Antigens - Screening of the serum samples for an IgG4 response with the test antigens was also performed. Figure 2 is a set of graphs of the IgG4 responses. While two of the high responding samples from the IgG analysis (sera 171 and 178) remain identifiable as high responders in the IgG4 screen, the remainder of the sera exhibit very low responses. This may indicate that the elevated absorbance levels correlate with the immunoglobulin isotype. Figure 3 is a graphic comparison of the specific IgG and IgG4 responses for those sera with IgG responses ≥ the mean plus the standard deviation of the mean for the total study population using both c55 and c56 as the test antigens. It is noteworthy that serum 178 is the only serum with a response value ≥ the mean plus twice the standard deviation of the mean for the test population. Table 2 also includes a compilation of those sera that exhibit IgG4 responses either ≥ the mean plus the standard deviation (stdev) (+) for the individual test antigen or ≥ the mean plus twice the standard deviation (2stdev) (++) for the individual test antigen.

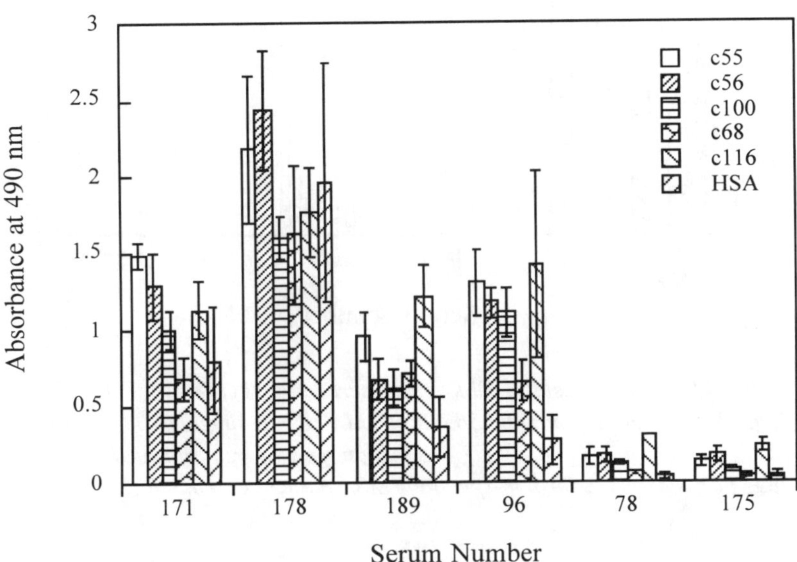

Figure 1- *IgG Screening Results. ELISA sera screen for IgG using TDI-HSA conjugate 55 (c55), TDI-HSA conjugate 56 (c56), TMA-HSA conjugate 100 (c100), MDI-HSA conjugate 68 (c68), soluble Rye Grass Allergen (c116) and HSA as test antigens were performed. All responses have been corrected for non-specific ELISA plate background.*

Concentration Normalization - Further analysis of the IgG response of sera to c56 was performed to determine whether the variability and high responses of the control sera to the TDI conjugates was related to the total IgG content of the test sera. To address this question, individual serum responses were divided by the total IgG concentration of the relevant sample. These "normalized" response values were then analyzed for the correlation to the absorbance values before correction for IgG concentration. A correlation coefficient (r^2) of 0.92 suggests that total IgG concentration does not account for the variable responses detected.

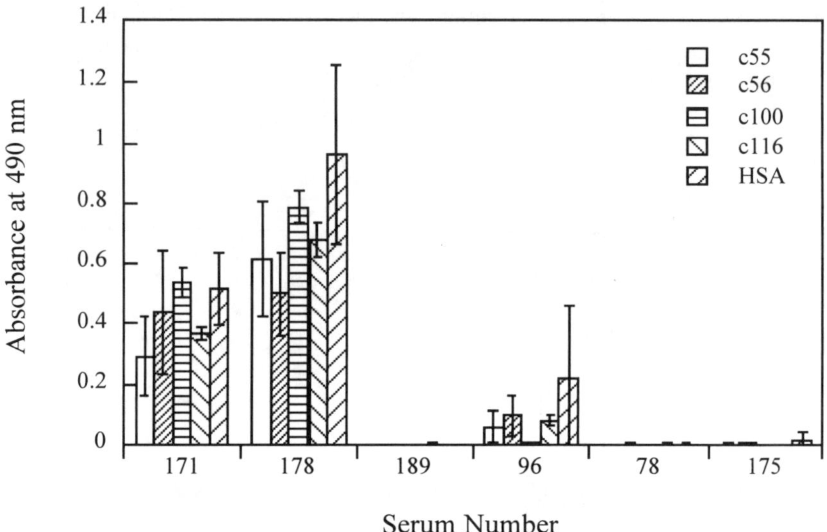

Figure 2 - *IgG4 Screening Results. ELISA sera screen for IgG4 using TDI-HSA conjugate 55 (c55), TDI-HSA conjugate 56 (c56), TMA-HSA conjugate 100 (c100), soluble Rye Grass Allergen (c116) and HSA as test antigens were performed. All responses have been corrected for non-specific ELISA plate background.*

Effect of Blocking Agent - Evaluation of the blocking reagent was performed to determine the possible effect on the background response level. Figure 4 is a graph of the comparison between results obtained using an 1% nonfat, dried milk solution or a 1% BSA blocking solution on the 96-well plates. All other conditions of the ELISA remained constant for these comparisons. Using BSA as the blocking agent, the background response level was reduced and only 2 samples (sera 80 and 178) indicated absorbance levels ≥ the mean plus the standard deviation of the mean for the group tested.

Specificity of Antibody Detection - To further test the specificity of the control sera responses observed, inhibition assays were conducted on all of the sera in the elevated response group (Table 2). Serum 152 from an TDI-exposed asthmatic individual, as determined by specific inhalation challenge, was used as a positive control (Figure 5A). Only one serum sample from the high response group (Serum #178, Figure 5B) showed specific inhibition with homologous test antigens. All the other sera demonstrated no inhibition by any of the test antigens.

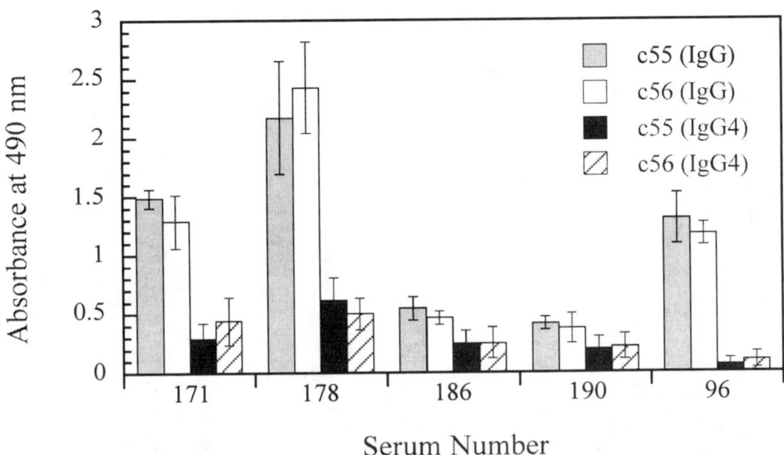

Figure 3 - *Comparison of IgG and IgG4 Responses. A comparison of IgG and IgG4 responses in ELISA with conjugate c55 and conjugate c56 as the test antigens is plotted. Data for all serum samples for which their IgG or IgG4 response to either c55 or c56 was ≥ the mean plus one standard deviation of the mean for the corresponding isotype (Table 2) are represented.*

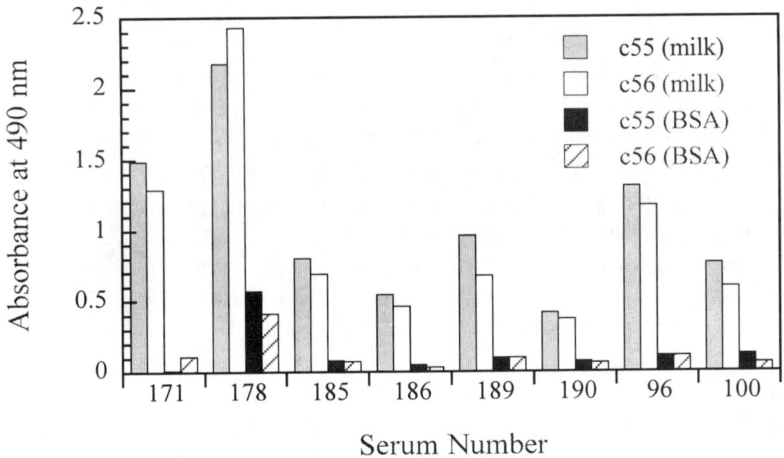

Figure 4 - *Comparison of the Effect of Blocking Agent. A comparison of 1% nonfat dried milk (MBS) and 1% BSA as blocking solutions in the ELISA with conjugates c55 and c56 as the test antigens is plotted. Data for all serum samples for which their IgG response to any of the test antigens was ≥ the mean plus one standard deviation of the mean using 1% milk as blocking agent are represented.*

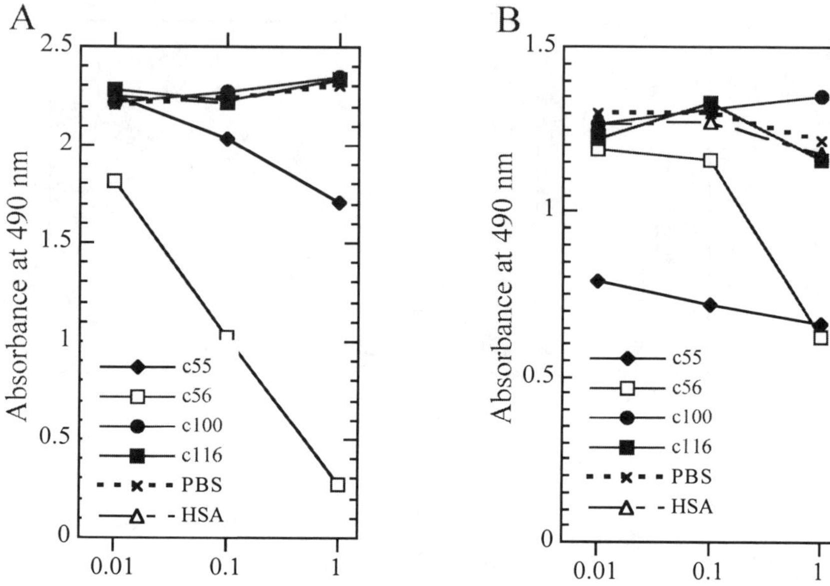

Relative Inhibitor Concentration

Figure 5 - *Determination of Specificity of Binding. Inhibition assays were performed on all sera for which their IgG or IgG4 response was ≥. The mean plus one standard deviation from the mean for the corresponding immunoglobulin isotype. Three serial dilutions of inhibitor were used in each case. Inhibitors tested were TDI-HSA (c55) (filled diamonds), TDI-HSA (c56) (open squares), TMA-HSA (c100) (filled circles), HSA (open triangles), and ryegrass (c116) (filled squares). Conjugate 56 was immobilized on the plate for each assay. Serum 152 (A) from a SIC-positive, TDI-exposed individual was used as a positive control, demonstrating inhibition with c55 and c56. Of the other sera examined, only serum 178 (B) showed specific inhibition with c55 and c56. None other conjugates showed inhibition.*

Discussion

The etiology of diisocyanate asthma has been debated for many years primarily because it is a complex disease process but also due to the lack of consistent correlation between specific antibody levels and proven or suspected disease state. A great deal of effort has been spent on the characterization of the associated immune response. The current study was initiated to further refine our understanding of the antibody test system and result interpretation with particular focus on general population responses. The analysis of the background reactivity in immunologic testing, particularly in reference to diisocyanate antibody screening, has not been extensively reported in the literature. In fact, many individualized methods of positive result classification have been implemented and for several published studies, the control population size is often very limited and/or not well defined. Our previous work has demonstrated that even when testing serum samples from individuals with no known exposure to isocyanates, some high-level antibody responses were detected with isocyanate conjugates. In addition, a population study evaluating possible environmental exposure has found individuals with elevated antibody levels independent of known exposure or disease symptomology [18]. Understanding the screening background and defining the control level of response is absolutely critical in the interpretation of diisocyanate antibody data. This is especially true in the case of TDI-associated disease since the detection of a meaningful absorbance reading above the background average (i.e., signal to noise ratio) is typically lower than the ratios observed for other diisocyanates such as MDI or HDI. The differential response levels detected in cases of TDI exposure necessitate a higher sensitivity in antibody screening methodologies without compromising specificity.

This study was conducted to implement an ELISA screening methodology on serum samples from individuals with no known isocyanate exposure. In this group of 30 samples, one sera (#178) was identified through IgG screening using a broad spectrum of test antigens including diisocyanate conjugates, a TMA conjugate, and ryegrass antigen (Figure 1, Table 2) as being ≥ 2 standard deviations above the mean for each conjugate tested. Using a cutoff criteria of $\geq$ the mean plus one standard deviation, 6 serum samples were classified as elevated responders (Table 2). Response to unmodified HSA was also evaluated and a similar pattern was observed. HSA reactivity has been recognized in other studies and in some cases has been corrected for through simple subtraction or application of complex algorithms. In this study, both test antigen and HSA responses are presented for direct comparison (Figures 1 and 2). Total IgG concentrations were also determined for each sample to analyze the effect variable IgG concentration may have on the background binding. The resulting absorbance per mg of IgG was found to correlate directly to the uncorrected response indicating that total IgG concentration did not interfere with the assay under the conditions tested.

In a previous study we demonstrated an enhanced selectivity in samples from a TDI-induced asthmatic population through the use of IgG4 isotype analysis [15]. To test whether the specific isotype, IgG4, could better define background response levels, similar screening was performed on this non-isocyanate-exposed population. The IgG4 testing resulted in the classification of two of the thirty control-samples as high responders (2 standard deviations above the mean, Table 2). In addition, a total of 4 samples (Table 2) met the criteria for elevated response ($\geq$ mean + standard deviation). Thus, under the assay conditions for this general population study, only minimal improvement in selectivity using IgG4 screening was observed.

Further refinement of the sample classification was obtained through specific and non-specific inhibition. All binding was determined to be non-specific except for serum 178 that demonstrated specific inhibition with diisocyanate antigens as illustrated in Figure 5. While this individual may have been exposed to isocyanates in a non-occupational setting, no asthmatic symptoms were reported and thus the response remains classified as a false positive.

In summary, the results of this study have illustrated an improved strategy for the identification of false positives in a non-isocyanate-exposed population. This strategy involves the use of IgG4 isotype screening and specific inhibition testing. This is particularly important in cases where the signal to noise ratio of the antibody response is low. In the cases of MDI and HDI induced asthma [4], the antibody response levels are typically much higher than those observed in TDI-induced asthmatics and therefore, true positives are more easily distinguishable. It is hoped that through a better understanding of the assay and control group responses, the detection of specific diisocyanate induced antibodies and subsequent diagnoses can be improved.

References

[1] Baur X. and Fruhmann G., "Specific IgE Antibodies in Patients with Isocyanate Asthma." *Chest,* Vol. 808, 1981, pp. 73-76.

[2] Butcher, B. T., O'Neil, C. E., Reed, M. E. and Salvaggio, J. E., "Radioallergosorbent Testing of Toluene Diisocyanate-Reactive Individuals Using p-tolyl Isocyanate Antigen" Journal *of Allergy and Clinical Immunology,* Vol. 66, 1980, pp. 213-216.

[3] Carter, A., Grammar, L., Malo, J. -L., Lager, F., Ghetto, H., Harris, K. and Patterson, R., "Specific serum antibodies against isocyanates: Association with occupational asthma". *Journal of Allergy and Clinical Immunology,* Vol. 84, 1989, pp. 507-514.

[4] Grammer, L. C., Harris, K. E., Malo, J.-L., Cartier, A. and Patterson, R., "The use of an immunoassay index for antibodies against isocyanate human protein conjugates and application to human isocyanate disease" *Journal of Allergy and Clinical Immunology,* Vol. 86, 1990, pp. 94-98.

[5] Karol, M., "Study of guinea pig and human antibodies to toluene diisocyanate". *American Review of Respiratory Diseases,* Vol. 122, 1980, pp. 965-970.

[6] Karol M. H., and Alane Y., "Antigens Which Detect IgE Antibodies in Workers Sensitive to Toluene Diisocyanate," *Clinical Allergy,* Vol. 10, 1980, pp. 101-109.

[7] Keskinen, H., Tupasela, U. and Nordman, H., "Experiences of Specific IgE in Asthma Due to Diisocyanates," *Clinical Allergy,* Vol. 18, 1988, pp. 597-604.

[8] Pezzini, A., Riviera, A., Paggiaro, P., Spiazzi, A., Gerosa, F., Filieri, M., Toma, G. and Tridente, G., "Specific IgE Antibodies in Twenty-eight Workers with

Diisocyanate Induced Bronchial Asthma," *Clinical Allergy*, Vol. 14, 1984, pp. 453-461.

[9] Banks, D. E., Butcher, B. T. and Salvaggio, J. E., "Isocyanate Induced Respiratory Disease," *Annals Allergy*, Vol. 57, 1986, pp. 389-396.

[10] Bernstein, I. L., "Isocyanate Induced Pulmonary Diseases: A Current Perspective," *Journal of Allergy and Clinical Immunology*, Vol. 70, 1982, pp. 24-31.

[11] Bernstein, I. L., Chan-Yeung, M., Malo, J.-L. and Bernstein, D. l., *Asthma in the Workplace*, Marcel Dekker, Inc., New York, 1993

[12] Mapp, C. E., Saetta, M., Maestrelli, P., Stefano, A. D., Chitano, P., Boschetto, P., Ciaccia, A. and Fabbri, L. M., "Mechanisms and Pathology of Occupational Asthma," *European. Respiratory Journal,* Vol. 7, 1994, pp. 544-554.

[13] Patterson, R., Hargreave, F. E., Grammer, L. C., Harris, K. E. and Dolovich, J., "Toluene Diisocyanate Respiratory Reactions: Reassessment of the Problem," *International Archives of Allergy and Applied Immunology*, Vol. 84, 1987, pp. 93-100.

[14] Brown, W. E., Green, A. H. Cedel, T. E. and Cairns, J., "Biochemistry of Protein-Isocyanate Interactions: A Comparison of the Effects of Aryl vs Alkyl Isocyanates," *Environmental Health Perspectives*, Vol. 72, 1987, pp. 5-11.

[15] Kennedy, A. L. and Brown, W. E., "Correlation of Diisocyanate Conjugate Immunologic Response and Clinical Diagnosis," 2000 (manuscript in preparation).

[16] Bollag, Daniel M., and Edelstein, Stuart J., *Protein Methods*, Wiley-Liss, Inc.. 1991.

[17] Engrall, E. and Perlman, P., "Enzyme-linked Immunosorbent Assay (ELISA): Quantitative Assessment of Immunoglobulin," *Immunochemistry*, Vol.. 8, 1971, pp. 871-879.

[18] Orloff, K. G., Batts-Osborne, D., Kilgus, T., Metcalf, S. and Cooper, M., "Antibodies to Toluene Diisocyanate in an Environmentally Exposed Population," *Environmental Health Perspectives*, Vol. 106, 1998, pp. 665-666.

Wm. Wesley Norton,[1] and Venkatram Dharmarajan[2]

Field Evaluation of a Gravimetric Sampling Method as a Screening Tool for the Monitoring of Airborne Isocyanates in Paint-Spray Operations

---

Reference: Norton W.W. and Dharmarajan, V., **"Field Evaluation of a Gravimetric Sampling Method as a Screening Tool for the Monitoring of Airborne Isocyanates in Paint-Spray Operations"**, *Isocyanates: Sampling, Analysis, and Health Effects, ASTM STP 1408*, J. Lesage, I. D. DeGraff, and R.S. Danchik, Eds., American Society for Testing and Materials, West Conshohocken, PA, 2002.

Abstract: The industrial applications of polyurethane coatings have been steadily growing. The reaction of polyisocyanates to polyols is the basis for all polyurethane coatings. The Oregon State OSHA PEL for HDI-polyisocyanates is 0.5 mg/m^3 8-hour TWA and 1.0 mg/m^3 ceiling. The recommended impinger sampling method for HDI-polyisocyanates is cumbersome and potentially hazardous.

Previous comparisons of impinger versus filter sampling in paint spray environments have shown that the filters can underestimate the polyisocyanate concentration. However, a recent NIOSH study concluded that an upper limit for the isocyanate concentrations in a paint-spray environment could be measured/calculated by a gravimetric method.

In this study, a PVC-filter gravimetric method was compared to an impinger-sampling method for measuring isocyanate concentrations during spray painting of automobiles. Seven side-by-side impinger and gravimetric sample sets were collected inside a custom-made chamber from a 2-gal plastic bottle. Each set consisting of four impingers and four filter cassettes with the same inlet orientation was mounted symmetrically inside the chamber. Tygon® tubing passing through the base connected the samplers to battery-operated pumps outside. Additionally, a vacuum pump connected to five holes at the base permitted the paint spray to be drawn into the chamber at isokinetic velocity.

Gravimetric samples were weighed with a precision analytical balance. Impinger samples were analyzed for isocyanates by a standard HPLC/UV method. The gravimetric weights were converted to isocyanate weights using a factor based on the paint formulation. The average isocyanate concentrations in mg/m^3 by the two methods were

---

[1] Senior Industrial Hygienist, Worldwide Facilities Group-Chemical Risk Management, General Motors Corporation, 1500 East Route A, Wentzville, MO 63385.

[2] HES Principal, Corporate Industrial Hygiene Department, Bayer Corporation, 100 Bayer Road, Pittsburgh, PA 15205.

statistically compared. The average ratio of gravimetric measurements to impinger measurements was 1.06 ± 0.15 % for n = 6 (total 48 samples). The gravimetric isocyanate concentrations are the theoretical maximums for the paint atmosphere sampled, whereas, the impinger isocyanate concentrations are the true in-situ values. The predictable correlation between the two methods suggests that the gravimetric method could serve as a screening tool for monitoring isocyanates in validated paint atmospheres.

Keywords: isocyanates, diisocyanates, polyisocyanates, industrial hygiene, polyurethane paint spray environment, air sampling, gravimetry, method evaluation, field validation, field comparison, impinger sampling

Introduction

Polyurethane coatings are widely used in automotive, aerospace, furniture and appliance industries. The basis of all polyurethane coatings is the reaction of an isocyanate with polyol to produce polyurethane. Aliphatic and aromatic polyisocyanates are the primary raw materials used for these coatings. Coatings based on aliphatic polyisocyanates are particularly suitable for automobiles and airplanes because of their light stability and weatherability.

Potential health effects of diisocyanates are generally considered to include acute irritation, and with exposure to higher concentrations, sensitization [1,2]. An 8-hour time weighted average TLV® of 5ppb is recommended for most of the monomeric diisocyanates. At the present time there are no federal OSHA, NIOSH or ACGIH recommended exposure limits for polyisocyanates; however, the Oregon OSHA occupational exposure standard is an 8-hr TWA of 0.5 mg/m^3 and a ceiling limit of 1 mg/m^3 for HDI-polyisocyanates. Bayer Corporation has established a Manufacturer's Guideline Limit (MGL) of 1.0 mg/m^3 as a short-term exposure limit (STEL-averaged over 15 minutes) [3]. The MGL also includes a 0.5 mg/m^3 TWA averaged over 8 hours. This TWA MGL of 0.5 mg/m^3 is 14.7 times higher than the TWA TLV for HDI monomer.

Exposure monitoring for isocyanates in spray-painting operations is a challenging problem. Direct-reading paper-tape monitors recommended for pure diisocyanate are not dependable for polyisocyanate and are unsuitable for use in spray-painting operations [4,5]. Isocyanate functional groups contained in particles or droplets are only partially available to react with the reagent in the tape (where as in an impinger, the solvent dissolves the particles and frees the functional groups allowing reaction with the derivatizing agent). In a spray paint environment, colored paint aerosol collected on the paper tape can interfere with the measurement of the optical reflectance of the colored stain produced by the reaction of the isocyanate with the reagent on the tape. Also, the paper tape monitors can be subject to large interferences from water vapor and oxidants (ozone, NO_2) in the sample area [6]. Sampling for isocyanates in the spray environments is best performed using indirect methods. In indirect methods, the samples are collected on a suitable medium, and the medium is shipped to a laboratory for analysis. The medium in which the isocyanate is collected is either treated with or contains a derivatizing agent. The high reactivity of isocyanates requires all the sampling methods to derivatize and stabilize the isocyanates during collection. Currently, high performance liquid chromatography (HPLC) is the most popular analytical technique for isocyanate analysis combined with UV, fluorescence, electrochemical, or mass-spectroscopic (MS) detection. The indirect isocyanate-sampling methods could be classified into two categories based on the collection techniques: (1) impinger methods, where isocyanates are collected in solutions with dissolved derivatizing reagent and (2) solvent free methods, where the isocyanates are collected on a dry, reagent-coated solid-sorbent. A reagent coated, binder-free, glass-fiber filter is the most commonly used substrate for the solvent free methods. Several impinger and coated-filter methods using a variety of derivatizing agents and solvents have been reported in the scientific literature and some of these methods have been adopted as reference methods by governmental authorities [7-16]. Several studies have compared impinger to coated-filter sampling methods for the measurement of monomeric and polyisocyanates in paint spray environments [17-24]. Most of these studies show that the filters compared to the impinger methods underestimated the isocyanate concentration. An exception to this is the 1998 study conducted jointly by the US Brooks Airforce base (BAFB), NIOSH, and Institut de Recherché en Santé et en Sécurité du Travail du Quebec (IRSST, Quebec, Canada) [23,24]. The BAFB/NIOSH/IRSST study, which evaluated selected impinger and coated filter methods in an isocyanate-based paint spray operation, showed that the dual-filter method [15], overestimated the polymeric isocyanate concentrations compared to the impinger methods.

In the same study [23,24], BAFB/NIOSH/IRSST compared a simple gravimetric filter method to the conventional filter and impinger methods based on HPLC analysis. In the gravimetric study, the poly vinyl chloride (PVC) filters were used to collect all non-volatile aerosols in the air including polyisocyanates, paint pigments, and paint additives. The aerosolized solvents collected by this method evaporate during sampling and storage. The filters were weighed until a constant weight was obtained to ensure solvent evaporation. The gravimetric weight was corrected to account for the actual polyisocyanate content of the paint. The assumption was made that the particulate collected on the filter will have the same ratio of polyisocyanate. The corrected polyisocyanate weight was reported in mg/m^3 units, using the volume of air sampled. The study compared the gravimetric polyisocyanate concentration to the total reactive isocyanate group (TRIG) concentration analytically determined by various isocyanate-specific methods [6,8,13,15]. In 50 of the 55 sets of comparisons, including personal and area samples, the gravimetric method always gave the highest calculated concentration compared to the other methods. In the BAFB/NIOSH/IRSST study, the area samples were collected by mounting the samplers on the chest of a mannequin. The personal samples were collected on the left and right sides of the worker's breathing zone. No special precautions were taken to minimize the effect of wind currents, eddy currents, and air turbulence in the comparison measurements. Nevertheless, the gravimetric measurements were consistent enough to hypothesize that the method could be used as a simple and inexpensive screening tool for polyisocyanate exposure monitoring.

There was significant variability in the results between gravimetric and impinger methods in the BAFB/NIOSH/IRSST study. In some cases the gravimetric results were 100 times greater than the impinger values. The authors believe that the variability was due to poor study design. Special precautions were not taken to ensure that the comparison samples were collecting the same environment. In this study extraordinary measures were taken to ensure that the two methods compared were in fact sampling the same paint spray environment. The study was designed to test the accuracy of prediction of airborne polyisocyanate concentration by a gravimetric method when the gravimetric result was corrected by the percent polyisocyanates in the paint system. The gravimetric method offers considerable advantages over the impinger method in ease of use, safety, and cost. The primary aim of the study was to develop a rapid screening method to identify work areas in and around spray operations, where the exposure potential to isocyanate aerosols exists. The study was conducted in isocyanate-based paint spray operations, in an automobile manufacturing plant. This method is not intended for use in non-spray application of isocyanates where significant levels of monomer may exist.

Experimental

Materials and Methods

High Performance Liquid Chromatography (HPLC) Analysis of Polyisocyanates - Bayer Corporate Industrial Hygiene Laboratory (BCIHL), Pittsburgh, PA, supplied the N-(4-nitrobenzyl)-propylamine (nitro-reagent) impinger absorber solution (2×10^{-4} M in toluene). The impinger samples were analyzed by the AIHA-accredited BCIHL by BCIHL Method 1.4.4. Method 1.4.4 was adapted from OSHA Method 18 [*10, 11*]. The major difference between OSHA Method 18 and the Bayer Method 1.4.4 is in sample collection. The OSHA Method uses a bubbler with fritted glass inlet at 1L/min flow rate, and the Bayer method uses a standard midget impinger at 1.7 L/min flow rate for sample collection. The OSHA 18 Method is used primarily for vapor collection. Bayer Method 1.4.4 is a better method for aerosol collection. The derivative was analyzed by HPLC with a Hewlett-Packard Series II, 1090 Liquid Chromatograph with HP-1050 variable wavelength UV detector at 254 nm. The analytical column used was 5 μm pore size, C-8, Phenomenex LUNA, packed in 10-cm X 4.6-mm ID, stainless steel column. Flow rate was 1.5 mL/min. The mobile phase solvents were: Pump A = Acetonitrile, Pump B = Buffer (1-% triethylamine in water adjusted to pH 3 with phosphoric acid). The injection volume was 20 μL. The limits of quantitation were 0.1 μg/sample for monomers and 1.4 μg/sample for polyisocyanates.

Gravimetric Analysis of Polyisocyanates - PPG Industries, Inc., industrial hygiene laboratory in Allison Park, PA, supplied the pre-weighed 37-mm PVC filters for the gravimetric samples. The samples were post weighed using the same balance. A Cahn microbalance Model M-31 was used for weighing filters. The microbalance is precise to 0.0005 mg. Limit of quantitation for the laboratory is 1.4 μg per sample. Samples were collected at a flow rate of 2.0 L/min. Gravimetric results were reported as concentration of total solids. Results were adjusted for percent of isocyanates in total solids using information provided by the paint manufacturer as described in the Results and Discussion section.

Study Design

The objective of this study was to concurrently sample the paint overspray with impingers and the gravimetric filters during the painting of automobiles, analyze the samples by the recommended procedures, and compare the results. One of the prime criteria in a rigorous side-by-side comparison study is that the two methods collect statistically comparable samples. This concern was addressed by conducting the side-by-side sampling inside a specially constructed chamber. This specially constructed chamber by design ensured that a representative spray environment from the spray booth was uniformly introduced into the chamber. The study design assured that every sampler inside the chamber sampled the same paint-spray atmosphere unaffected by wind drafts and/or unexpected turbulence.

Field-Comparison Test Chamber

A round 2-gal polypropylene bottle with 1.5"-id opening and 7.5"-id body served as the chamber. The bottom of the bottle was cut out, and the bottle was mounted upright on a custom-made 2" thick wooden base. The bottle was then sealed to the base with polyethylene tape (see Figure 1A & 1B). Four blind holes (1"-od x 1.5"-deep) were drilled symmetrically along the circumference of a 2.5" radius circle in the wood base to hold the impingers. For the gravimetric filters, four 0.25"-od holes were drilled on the same circle midway between the impinger positions. Upright stainless steel (ss) tubes (0.25"-od) were inserted through these 4 holes, so that, when the gravimetric filter cassettes were attached to these tubes the filter-cassette inlets were at the same height as the impinger inlets. The samplers were connected to battery-operated pumps placed outside the bottle via 0.25"-id Tygon™ tubing. The tubing exited the chamber through airtight holes in the wooden base. Additionally, five 0.5"-od holes were drilled in the base; one in the center and four at the periphery at right angles. Copper tubes (0.5"-od) were inserted into these holes from the bottom such that the tube ends were flush with the base floor. The four peripheral copper tubes were bent and connected centrally to a manifold outside, and below the wooden base. The fifth copper tube in the center of the base was connected directly to the manifold. The manifold exit was connected to an exhaust vacuum/pressure pump (see Figure 1a) via thick-rubber hose through a needle valve. The needle valve controlled the airflow into the bottle through the five openings at the base. The total airflow into the bottle, by the vacuum/pressure and the sampling pumps, was adjusted to achieve isokinetic velocity by matching the velocity to the downdraft velocity in the spray booth.

A custom-made PVC pipe (1.5" id x 24" long) was mounted vertically to the bottle inlet via the bottle cap and a PVC reducer union. This device was used to measure the air velocity into the bottle. A 3/8" hole drilled into the pipe 12" from the bottle inlet permitted insertion of a TSI -thermal anemometer probe for air velocity measurements. With all the eight battery-operated pumps and the vacuum/pressure pump running, the airflow into the bottle was adjusted using the needle valve and the thermal anemometer to match the downdraft velocity in the spray-booth. The PVC tube was removed before the experimental tests. The average spray booth velocity was approximately 70 feet per minute. For conveniently sampling at a desired location, the entire experimental set up (polypropylene bottle, wooden base, four impingers, four filters, and eight battery-operated pumps) was placed in a 20"x24" portable plastic tray. A long rubber hose (≈20 ft x 3/8") connected the exhaust manifold to the vacuum/pressure pump placed outside the spray booth. An in line jumbo charcoal trap was used to capture the paint spray and solvents entrained by the pumps thus protecting the pumps and personnel outside of the booth. Two isokinetic-sampling-bottle kits were constructed and used for the study. For every test run, four gravimetric filters and four

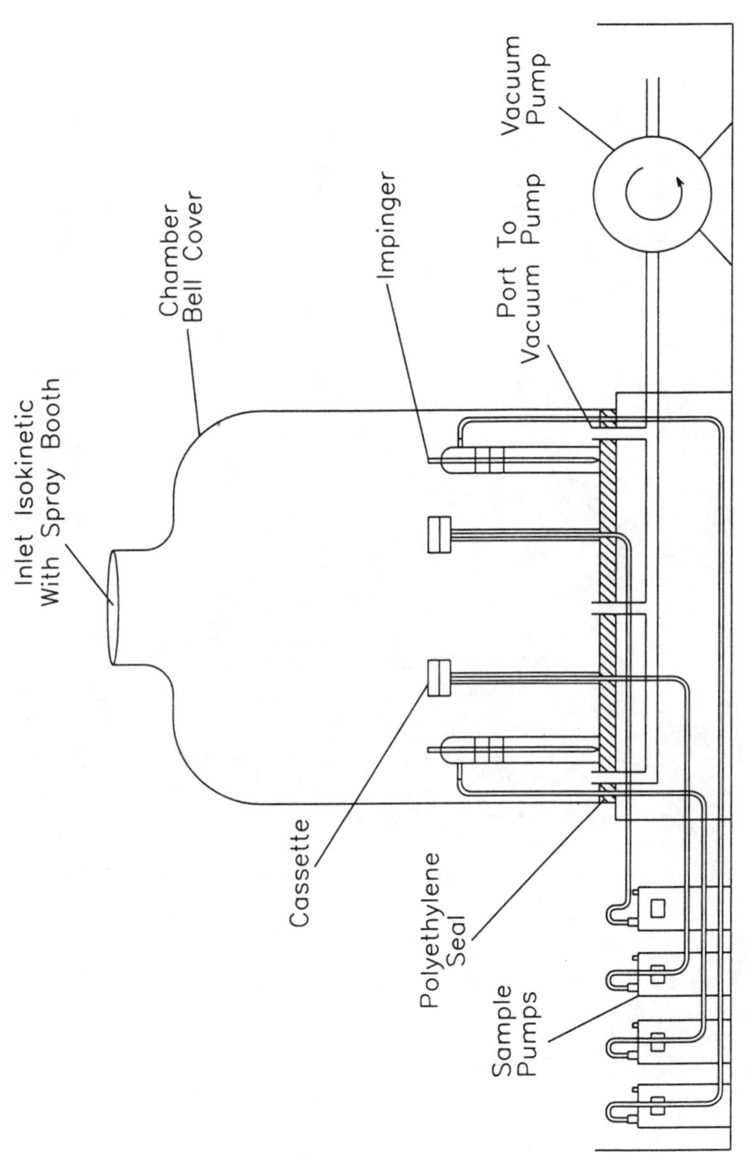

Figure 1A – Lateral View – Sample Apparatus

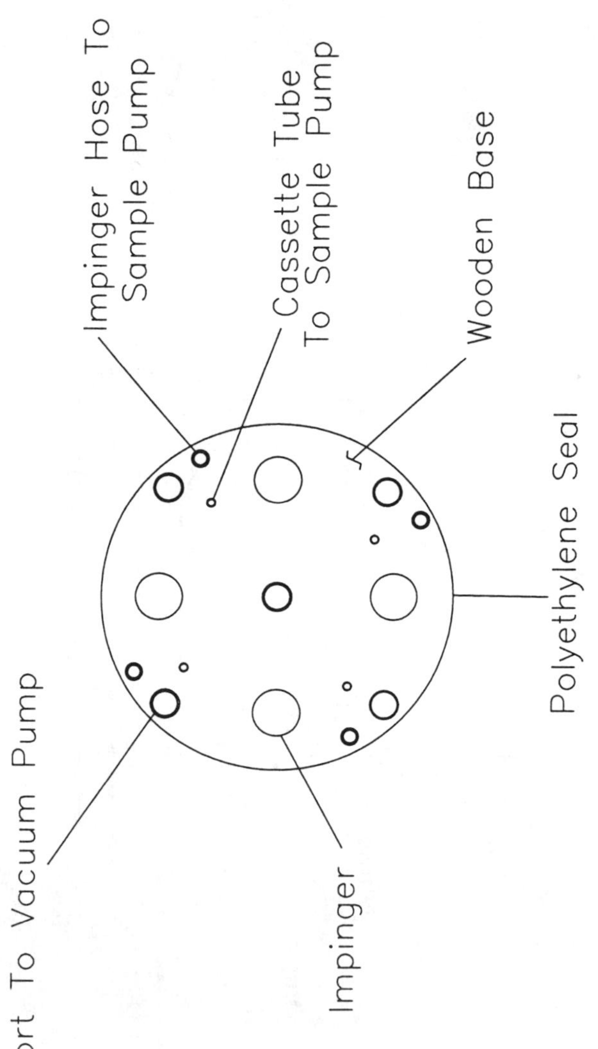

Figure 1B – Plan View – Sample Apparatus Base

impingers were symmetrically mounted inside the bottle with their inlets facing up at the same height.

Testing Procedure

The following sequence was followed for every sampling session.

(1) The polypropylene bottle was removed from the wooden base.
(2) Four midget impingers, each with 15-20 mL of fresh nitro-reagent, were placed in the receptacles provided. Four gravimetric filter cassettes were attached to the four SS ports facing up. The impinger and the filter cassettes were connected to the battery-operated pumps via the Tygon™ tubes connected to the appropriate outlets at the bottom of the wooden base.
(3) The impinger and the gravimetric-filter flows were calibrated to 1.7 L/min and 2.0 L/min, respectively, using an electronic soap-bubble calibrator.
(4) The plastic bottle was placed over the impingers and the filters. The PVC tube was attached to the bottle and the vacuum/pressure pump was connected to the exhaust manifold with the long rubber hose. The vacuum pump and the battery-operated pumps were turned on. The inlet velocity was checked with the thermal anemometer and adjusted to the desired isokinetic value using the needle valve.
(5) The pumps were turned off. The PVC tube was removed, the plastic bottle was also removed, and the impingers were wrapped in disposable Kwik-cold® ice packs with rubber bands to minimize solvent evaporation during the test period. The bottle was mounted again. The entire apparatus was placed at the target sampling location.
(6) All sampling pumps and the vacuum/pressure pump were turned on and the start time was recorded. After sampling for the pre-selected sample time the tray was brought out of the booth, the sampler pumps were turned off, and the time recorded. The sampling times were ≈50 - 70 minutes.
(7) Immediately after a sampling session, the filter cassettes were removed, sealed, and stored in a secure location at room temperature. The impinger solutions and rinses were transferred to 30-mL amber bottles and stored in a refrigerator at 0°C before shipping to BCIHL for analysis. The filter samples were shipped to PPG industrial hygiene laboratory for post-weighing.

Results and Discussion

The paint used for spraying the automobiles contained HDI and IPDI based polyisocyanate hardeners. Theoretical total isocyanate concentration was determined by factoring the mix ratio of the two-part paint (2 parts polyol to 1 part polyisocyanate hardener), the percent solids in the paint formula, and the percent isocyanate in the hardener. The actual paint composition is proprietary; however, values were provided by the paint manufacturer to establish a correction factor calculated from percent polyisocyanate in paint, two component mix ratio, and percent solids as shown in the following formula:

Isocyanate weight by   =   Gravimetric weight (mg) x % polyisocyanate in paint
the gravimetric method   x mix ratio / % solids

The isocyanate concentration in mg/m^3 by the gravimetric method was calculated using the volume of air sampled by the filter.

The impinger samples were analyzed for HDI and IPDI monomers and for HDI and IPDI polyisocyanates. The weights of the four species were summed to obtain the total weight of the isocyanates by the impinger method. In the impinger analytical results, the isocyanate weight was predominantly due to polyisocyanates. An average of 2.9% of the isocyanate weight was due to monomers (HDI+IPDI) in low concentration areas and an average of 0.5% in the high concentration areas. The impinger-isocyanate weights were converted to mg/m^3 units for comparison with the gravimetric method.

Seven sets of field comparison samples were collected, three in high concentration spray area and four in low concentration areas. Table 1 summarizes the average mg/m^3 and the standard deviation for each run by the gravimetric and the impinger methods.

Table 1 - *Comparison of Gravimetric to Impinger Sampling and Analysis Method for the Measurement of Polyisocyanates*

Exp. No.	Gravimetric Method Polyisocyanate Conc. Mg/m^3			Impinger Method Polyisocyanate Conc. mg/m3			Ratio[1] Gravimetry to Impinger
	N	Mean	1 SD	N	Mean	1SD	
1	4	5.72	1.07	4	4.35	0.72	1.32
2	4	11.50	2.25	4	9.27	0.53	1.23
3	4	4.76	0.36	4	4.62	0.72	1.03
4	4	≤0.19	NA[2]	4	≤.043[3]	0.03	NA
5	4	0.15	0.08	4	0.16	0.02	0.92
6	4	0.21	0.08	4	0.23	0.04	0.93
7	4	0.29	0.19	4	0.32	0.04	0.92

[1] The average ratio for all measurements, excluding experiment four is 1.06 ± 0.15 (n=6)
[2] In experiment 4, three of the four gravimetric sample weights were less than the blanks. Blank correction made those weights negative.
[3] In this set, for two of the 4 impinger samples, the IPDI-polyisocyanate values were less than the limit of quantitation (1.38 µg/sample) and in one of those two samples the HDI value was less than the LOQ of 0.1 µg/sample.

The average polyisocyanate impinger values were statistically compared to the average gravimetric values using paired t-test. The t-test evaluation result is shown graphically in Figure 2A. The ideal 1:1 correlation and the actual correlation lines with the 95% confidence limits are shown in the graph. The ideal correlation line is within the 95% confidence limits, which means the two averages are not significantly different at this confidence level. The 95% confidence limits intersect the gravimetry (X) axis at ≈ -0.48 and 1.6 mg/m^3 units, suggesting that the quantitation limit of the gravimetric method

Bivariate Fit of Impinger Method - mg/m3 By Gravimetric Method - mg/m3

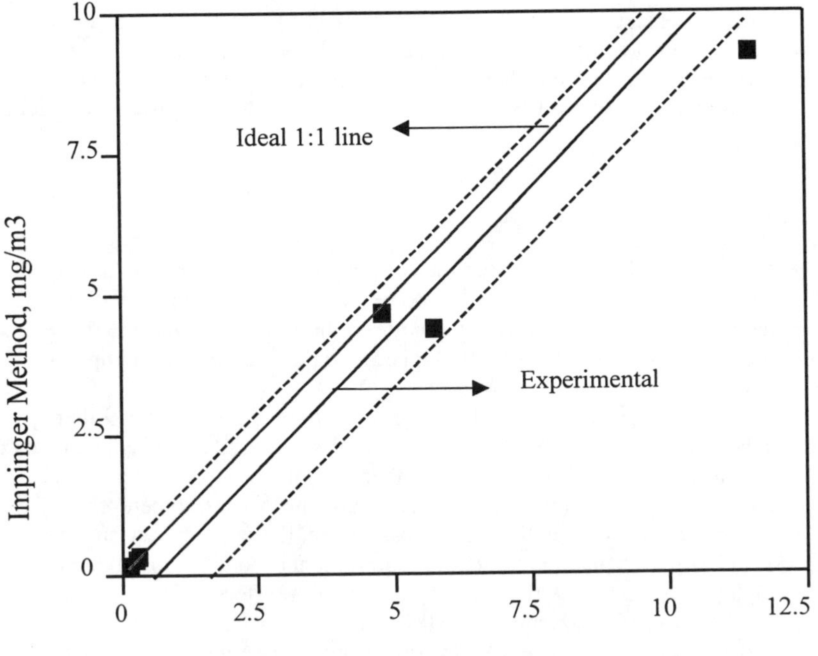

Paired T Test

Impinger Method, mg/m3 - Gravimetric Method, mg/m3

Mean Difference	-0.61333	Prob > |t|	0.1786
Std Error Dif	0.392162	Prob > t	0.9107
T Ratio	-1.56398	Prob < t	0.0893
DF	5		

Figure 2A Comparison of Gravimetric method to Impinger method
at high and low paint spray concentrations

is 1.6 mg/m^3, which is 3 times the recommended exposure limit of 0.5 mg/m^3 TWA. However, this is deceptive because the confidence limits are affected by the high concentrations. Therefore, the 16 comparison measurements at the low exposure areas were compared using the paired t-test. The results are shown in Figure 2B. The negative gravimetric results were assigned the value of zero. It is clear from the Figure 2B that the confidence limits intersect at ≈ - 0.075 and 0.03 mg/m^3, suggesting that the gravimetric results can be used confidently to measure levels of 0.2 mg/m^3 levels.

The authors believe that the excellent correlation between the impinger and gravimetric sample results is due to representative sample collection inside the specially designed chamber.

Conclusions

Results of this study indicate that gravimetric sampling can be used as a surrogate method to accurately measure and predict airborne polyisocyanate concentration.   There was good statistical correlation between the methods, however, the gravimetric method tended to produce values that were slightly higher than the corresponding impinger method at concentrations greater than 5 mg/m^3.

Gravimetric sampling offers many advantages over impinger sampling. Filter cassettes can be readily used for breathing zone samples, are easily handled, and are not subject to special shipping requirements. Impinger sampling requires the use of a toluene/ nitroreagent with flammable, toxic and volatile properties. Inherent to this method are risks to workers, potential breakage, spillage, frequent replenishment of reagent, special hazardous materials shipping requirements and difficulty in obtaining personal samples. Also, gravimetric sampling is more cost effective, and has faster turnaround time compared to the impinger/HPLC method.

Sampling time plays a significant role in comparing the two methods.   Due to evaporation of toluene/nitroreagent and the requirement to replenish the reagent, impinger sample times are frequently of relatively short duration. Gravimetric sample times can easily be full shift. However, the analytical limit of quantitation for the gravimetric method and the relatively low recommended exposure limit for polyisocyanates also make long sample periods necessary.

The advantages of the gravimetric method and predictable correlation between the two methods suggest that gravimetric sampling can serve as a surrogate sampling method and screening tool for monitoring polyisocyanates in work environments. Gravimetric measurement of total solids concentration adjusted by a correction factor (calculated from percent polyisocyanate in paint, two component mix ratio, and percent solids) provided by the paint manufacturer gives a good estimate of polyisocyanate concentration.

Surrogate Sampling Method

Polyisocyanate concentrations typically exceed the recommended exposure limit in spray zones of paint booths or paint areas. At higher concentrations (>5 mg/m^3) the gravimetric method slightly overestimates the polyisocyanate concentrations.

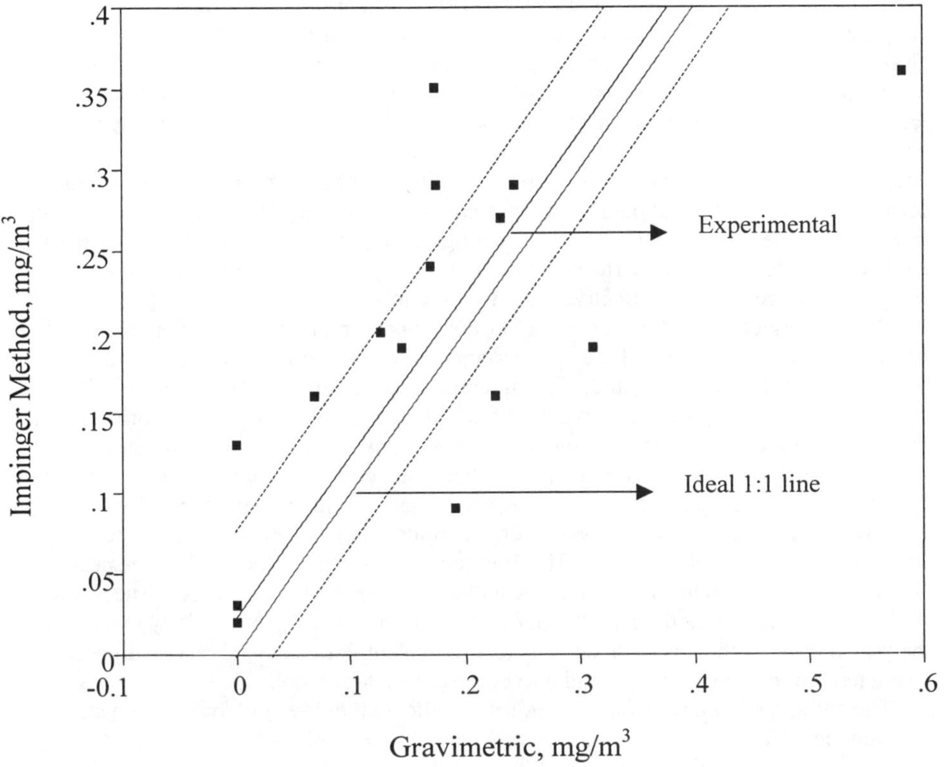

Paired T Test
Impinger, mg/m3 - Gravimetric, mg/m3

Mean Difference	0.022475	Prob > |t|	0.3948
Std Error Dif	0.025655	Prob > t	0.1974
T Ratio	0.876037	Prob < t	0.8026
DF	15		

Figure 2B   Comparison of Gravimetric method to Impinger method at low paint spray concentrations

Nevertheless, the adjusted gravimetric data will be sufficiently accurate to establish appropriate protection factors for respiratory protection.

Surrogate Screening Tool

Frequently, polyisocyanate monitoring is performed at the perimeter of spray booths or spray areas to confirm effectiveness of controls in containing paint aerosol. Gravimetric samples taken in areas expected to have air concentrations below the recommended exposure limit can be used as a screening tool. Adjusted gravimetric results of less than half the recommended limit of 0.5 mg/m^3 can be confidently used as confirmation of no overexposure. Best practice is to maintain exposure to polyisocyanates to the lowest feasible level. Adjusted gravimetric results greater than background levels (typical paint shop approximately 0.2 mg/m^3) would be followed with sampling for the specific polyisocyanates using the impinger method. The gravimetric method can also be used to perform sampling under supplied air hoods of workers in spray zones to confirm the effectiveness of protection.

Monitoring of polyisocyanates is a key component in protection of workers in paint spray operations. Selection of the appropriate method is important to ensure that all isocyanates present are measured. The high reactivity of isocyanates requires all the conventional sampling methods to derivatize and stabilize the isocyanates during collection. Impinger methods using derivatizing reagent are the most widely accepted method of sampling for isocyanate aerosol but are cumbersome, costly and potentially hazardous. PVC filter gravimetric sampling can be used as a surrogate sample method to reduce the need for impinger samples by adjusting results of total solids measured to polyisocyanate concentration as described above. (This method is not intended for use in non-spray application of isocyanates where significant levels of monomer may exist). The advantages of the gravimetric method make it easier and less costly to sample. A likely result of use of the gravimetric method as a surrogate is that more samples can be taken resulting in better characterization of exposure potential to polyisocyanate aerosol.

The authors recommend further studies to validate these results for use with significantly different paint formulations.

Acknowledgments

The authors thank Ms. Marla Kruth of PPG, Inc. for assisting with the gravimetric analysis, Mr. Joel C. Johnson, GM/UAW, IH Technician, for assistance with sample collection and Mr. Tom Frampton of Bayer Corporation for analyzing the HPLC samples.

References

[1] National Institute for Occupational Safety and Health (NIOSH): *Criteria for a Recommended Standard: Occupational Exposure to Diisocyanates*, NIOSH Publication No. 78-215, U.S. Department of Health and Human Services, Public Health Service, Centers for Disease Control and Prevention, Cincinnati, OH, 1978.

[2] National Institute for Occupational Safety and Health (NIOSH): *Pocket Guide to Chemical Hazards*, NIOSH Publication No. 90-117, U.S. Department of Health and Human Services, Public Health Service, Centers for Disease Control and Prevention, Cincinnati, OH, 1990.

[3] Bayer Corporation: Internal Report, Bayer Corporation, Pittsburgh, PA 15205-9741.

[4] MDA Paper tape monitors for several isocyanates, TDI, HDI, MDI and others, from MDA Scientific, a division of Zellweger Analytics, Inc., Lincolnshire, IL.

[5] GMD Paper tape monitors for several isocyanates, TDI, HDI, MDI and others, manufactured and distributed by Scott-Bacharach Company, Exton, PA.

[6] Gardner, C., and D'Arcy, J. B., "The Use of Statistical Techniques in the Performance Evaluation of Workplace Air Monitors and Their Application to the Development of a Paper-Tape Monitor for Hexamethylene Diisocyanate (HDI) with Minimal Cross Sensitivity to Water Vapor and Atmospheric Oxidants." *American Industrial Hygiene Conference and Exhibition*, May 19-23, 1997.

[7] NIOSH manual of Analytical Methods, 4th Edition, Peter M.Eller, Editor, U.S. Department of Health and Human Services, Public Health Service, Center for Disease Control and Prevention, National Institute for Occupational Safety and Health, Methods 5521, 5522, August 1994.

[8] Streicher, R. P., Arnold, J. E., Ernst, M. K., and Cooper, C. V., "Development of a Novel Derivatization Reagent for the Sampling and Analysis of Total Isocyanate Group in Air and Comparison of its Performance with that of Several Established Reagents" *American Industrial Hygiene Association Journal* 1996, 57, pp. 905-913.

[9] National Institute for Occupational Safety and Health (NIOSH), "Determination of Airborne Isocyanate Exposure" In: NIOSH Manual of Analytical Methods, Cassinelli, M.E and O'Connor, P.F., editors, 4th ed., 2nd supplement, DHHS(NIOSH) Publication No. 98-119, U.S. Department of Health and Human Services, Public Health Service, Centers for Disease Control and Prevention, NIOSH, Cincinnati, OH, 1998.

[10] Occupational Safety and Health Administration, OSHA Manual of Analytical Methods, Method No.18, Organic Methods Evaluation Branch, OSHA Analytical Laboratory, Salt Lake City, UT, February 1980.

[11] Bayer Corporation: Internal Report. Methods for the Sampling and Analysis of Airborne Isocyanates Method 1.44, October 2, 1997, Bayer Corporation, Pittsburgh, PA 15205-9741.

[12] Health and Safety Executive: MDHS 25/3, Methods for the Determination of Hazardous Substances: Organic Isocyanates in Air, Occupational Safety and Hygiene Laboratory, Health and Safety Executive, London, U.K. 1999.

[13] Occupational Safety and Health Administration, OSHA Manual of Analytical Methods, Method No. 42 for HDI and TDI, and Method No. 47 for MDI, Organic Methods Evaluation Branch, OSHA Analytical Laboratory, Salt Lake City, UT, February 1980.

[14] Tucker, S. P., and Arnold, J. E., "Sampling and Determination of 2,4-Bis(carbonylamino)toluene and 4,4'-Bis(carbonylamino)diphenylmathane in Air, *Analytical Chemistry*, 1982, 54, pp. 1137-1141.

[15] Lesage, J., Goyer, N., Desjardins, F. Vincent J.Y., Perrault, G., "Workers' Exposure to Isocyanates" *American Industrial Hygiene Association Journal*, 1992, 53, pp. 146-153..

[16] Czarnecki, B., "Polymeric-HDI Aerosol Sampling Efficiency Comparison: Impinger vs. ASA-coated Foam Sampler", Poster Session 302, Paper #353, American Industrial Hygiene Conference and Exposition, Atlanta, GA, May 1998.

[17] Maitre, A., Lepay, A., Perdix, A., Ohl, G., Boinay, P., Romazini, S., and Aubrun, J. C., " Comparison Between Solid Sampler and Impinger for Evaluation of Occupational Exposure to 1,6-Hexamethylene Diisocyanate Polyisocyanates During Spray Painting" *American Industrial Hygiene Association Journal*, 1996, 57, pp. 153-160.

[18] Rudzinski, W. E., Dahlquist, B., Svejda, S. A., Richardson, A., and Thomas, T. "Sampling and Analysis of Isocyanates in Spray-Painting Operations" *American Industrial Hygiene Association Journal*, 1995, 56, pp. 284-289.

[19] Levine, S. P., Hillig, K. J. D., Dharmarajan, V., Spence, M. W., and Baker, M. D., "Critical Review of Methods of Sampling, Analysis, and Monitoring for TDI and MDI" *American Industrial Hygiene Association Journal*, 1995, 56, pp. 581-589.

[20] Myer, H. E., O'Block, S.T., and Dharmarajan, V., " A Survey of Airborne HDI, HDI-based Polyisocyanate and Solvent Concentrations in Manufacture and Application of Polyurethane Coatings" *American Industrial Hygiene Association Journal*, 1993, 54, pp. 663-670.

[21] Czarnecki, B. and Hermes, B. J., "Polyisocyanate Sampling Using Coated-filter vs. Impinger Collection Systems" presented at the American Industrial Hygiene Conference and Exposition in Boston, MA. June 1992.

[22] Rosenberg, C. and Tuomi, T., "Airborne Isocyanates in Polyurethane Spray Painting: Determination and Respirator Efficiency" *American Industrial Hygiene Association Journal,* 1984, 45, pp. 117-121.

[23] England, E. C., Key-Schwartz, R., Carlton, G., and Lesage, J., " Comparison of Sampling Methods for 1,6-Hexamethylene Diisocyanate During Spray Finishing Operations" Poster Session Abstracts, American Industrial Hygiene Conference and Exposition 1998, Atlanta, GA.

[24] England, E. C., Key-Schwartz, R., Lesage, J., Carlton, G., Streicher, R., and Song, R., "Comparison of Sampling Methods for Monomer and Polyisocyanates of 1,6-Hexamethylene Diisocyanate During Spray Finishing Operations" *Applied Occupational and Environmental Hygiene*, 2000, 15, pp. 472-478.

Halet G. Poovey [1] and Roy J. Rando [1]

Workplace TRIG and Air-Purifying Respiratory Protection

Reference: Poovey, H. G. and Rando, R. J., **"Workplace TRIG and Air-Purifying Respiratory Protection,"** *Isocyanates: Sampling, Analysis, and Health Effects, ASTM STP 1408*, J. Lesage, I. D. Degraff, and R. S. Danchik, Eds., American Society for Testing and Materials, West Conshohocken, PA, 2002.

Abstract: Paired total and respirable particulate samples were collected in the breathing zone of 186 painters at five Air Force bases. Using the composition of the starting material to estimate total reactive isocyanate group (TRIG), exposure levels were 0.87 mg/M^3 (geometric mean) in the total fraction and 0.12 mg/M^3 in the respirable fraction with geometric standard deviations of 2.7 and 3.3, respectively. Dichotomous samplers specific for TRIG were used during the painting of a military vehicle and indicated 0.39 ± 0.15 mg/M^3 TRIG. This was 20 times the Health and Safety Executive's recommended time weighted average for TRIG. The TRIG levels seen in these studies indicate the need for personal protective equipment or additional engineering controls. Breakthrough studies with 1,6 hexamethylene diisocyanate (HDI) and HDI-biuret were conducted on a series of negative pressure air purifying respirator (APR) cartridges. Initial penetration of TRIG through the APR cartridges ranged from greater than 70% to less than 3% giving apparent protection factors of >1.5 and >33. These samples also showed that HDI was present in the aerosol fraction at levels significantly below its saturated vapor pressure.

Keywords: aerosols, isocyanate, respirators, spray painting, TRIG

---

[1] Research Assistant Professor and Associate Professor, respectively, Tulane University, School of Public Health & Tropical Medicine, Department of Environmental Health Sciences, 1430 Tulane Ave. - SL15, New Orleans, LA 70112.

Introduction

The efficacy of air purifying respirators (APR) for protection from isocyanate exposure has long been debated[1-2]. Support for the use of APRs comes from studies which show that monomeric isocyanates in vapor form are rapidly and effectively adsorbed by organic vapor cartridges[3]. There is additional support for the use of APRs from studies of paint overspray atmospheres showing that the PEL for the monomeric isocyanates is rarely exceeded. [4,5] However, the isocyanate monomers have very poor warning properties. With Occupational Safety and Health Administration (OSHA) permissible exposure limits (PEL) of 20 ppb for the regulated monomers and odor thresholds ranging from 50 ppb to 400 ppb, depending on the specific isocyanate, there is the potential for significant overexposure. However, in paint overspray atmospheres studies show that solvents with good warning properties penetrate more rapidly than do monomeric isocyanates[6]. It is argued that the solvents would therefore provide the adequate warning properties that had been required by NIOSH to protect the worker from excess exposure.

Official interpretations of OSHA regulations specifically banned the use of APR for protection from isocyanates. 1982 – *It is a violation of our standards to use a negative pressure paint spray respirator, whether approved or not, for protection against paint sprays containing isocyanates*[7]. 1987- *Air purifying respirators may not be used as a means of protecting employees overexposed to isocyanates*[8]. 1991 – *Positive pressure air-line respirators are the only approved respirators for employees who are exposed to isocyanates, regardless if an overexposure exists or not*[9].   However, more recent interpretations of the respiratory protection standard opened the door for their use. 1996 –*OSHA can only require the use of respiratory protection where we can document that an overexposure has or is likely to occur. In the case of spray painting in autobody shops, our sampling data from this industry has found virtually no overexposure to isocyanates. Workers could currently wear a half mask respirator with organic vapor cartridges and be within our requirements provided the employees were not exposed to isocyanates above our permissible exposure limits*[10]. In 1998 the revised OSHA respiratory protection standard allowed the use of APR for protection against isocyanates if an appropriate change out schedule were developed.

This debate has grown to include the potential health effects of isocyanate polymers. Animal models have indicated HDI-Biuret to be a potent pulmonary irritant, and have suggested an allowable exposure level of about 0.5 mg/M^3[11]. This figure has been adopted as a recommended exposure guideline by isocyanate manufacturers and the Oregon state OSHA[12]. There are an increasing number of case reports in the literature linking exposure to polyisocyanates from spray painting to various pulmonary diseases, including asthma [13-15] and hypersensitivity pneumonitis[16]. There is also a demonstrated association between exposure to HDI and its polymers to increased annual lung function decline[17,18].

Evidence of polymeric isocyanates affecting health in the same manner as monomers has led to the suggestion of treating all isocyanates together as total reactive isocyanate group (TRIG). TRIG consists essentially of all free isocyanate chemical groups present in the work place environment including monomeric, polymeric, and partially reacted isocyanates. The Health and Safety Executive in the United Kingdom has a recommended 8-hour TWA of 0.02 mg/M^3 with a 10-minute TWA of 0.07 mg/M^3 for TRIG. On a TRIG basis this standard is comparable to the Oregon State OSHA standard for Polymeric HDI, 0.05 mg/M^3. This paper will present the results of workplace exposure assessments and respirator cartridge testing for HDI-derived TRIG in simulated and real spray painting environments.

Materials and Methods

For the occupational exposure assessment, total and respirable particulate samples were collected via personal monitoring. Nine sets of samples were collected at five sites over a two-year period. Paired total and respirable particulate samples were collected in the breathing zone of 186 painters in paint shops and painting hangars. Particulate mass levels were determined gravimetrically using pre-weighed 25 millimeter Teflon filters, 1 µM pore size (Millipore FA). Both total and respirable samples were collected concurrently in the breathing zone of the painter while actively painting. Total aerosol samples were collected in open-faced polystyrene cassettes with a flow of 2 L/min. Respirable samples utilized a cyclone pre-separator (SKC, Model 225-01-01) to remove the non-respirable fractions. These samples were collected at a flow rate of 1.9 L/min. Samples were pre- and post- weighed after humidity conditioning over saturated sodium dichromate. Material Safety Data Sheets (MSDS) were collected for the paints being used at the time of sampling. These sheets provided information on the proportions of components to be mixed and the composition of the components. The maximum theoretical TRIG concentration was calculated from the composition of the starting materials.

In a second occupational exposure assessment the Tulane dichotomous sampler was used to measure vapor and condensed phase TRIG in a representative workplace atmosphere. The dichotomous sampler consists of a cyclone inlet for collection of non-respirable aerosols, followed by an annular diffusional denuder tube for collection of vapor, and backed up by a treated filter for collection of respirable aerosol. The samplers were operated at a flow rate of 2.0 L/min which resulted in an inlet cyclone cut diameter of 3.5 µm. The denuder and inlet are constructed from aluminum, glass, stainless steel, and Teflon and are commercially available from University Research Glassware (Carrsboro, NC). The denuders and back up filter were coated with MAMA, Aldrich catalog # 27,008-3 and tributylphosphate (TBP), Aldrich catalog # 24,049-4 for the collection of TRIG. Area sampling was conducted in a paint spray booth during mixing of the two part polyurethane paint, application of the paint, and cleanup and drying. The paint was based on HDI. A total of ten samples wascollected. The samples were analyzed as previously described[19].

Breakthrough studies were conducted on three cartridge configurations: 1) organic vapor cartridge, North (Cranston, RI) part # 7500-1 (OV); 2) organic vapor cartridge, North part # 7500-1 with paint spray pre-filter, North part # 7500-10 (OV/PP); and 3) organic vapor cartridge with high efficiency filter, North part # 7500-81 (OV/HE).

Cartridges were used as received. No pre-conditioning of the cartridges was performed. All cartridges were tested at a constant flow of 27 L/min. This rate is equivalent to one half the minute flow of a man under heavy working conditions, 830 kg-m/min. [20] Cartridges from a dual cartridge respirator were used in the study. Since only half the flow would pass through a given cartridge, the minute flow rate was divided by two. The chamber operated under positive pressure, and was flushed at a flow rate of about 2800 L/min. with room air, resulting in an average flow velocity of 30 m/min. in the sampling cross-section. Test atmosphere and dilution air were mixed by passing through a series of perforated plate diffusers. The atmosphere then passed through a honeycomb flow straightener (tubular cells of 28-mm diameter and 155-mm length) before entering the sampling zone. The chamber was placed in a walk in fume hood during use. The respirator cartridge ports in the aerosol chamber consisted of a section of a North full face respirator lens with inlet valve, seals and fittings, as would normally be seen in an intact respirator. The lens section was riveted around a 3.2 cm diameter opening in the wall of the chamber, and sealed with silicone sealant. The port was connected to a sampling train and the flow pump, with a section of 3.8 cm schedule 40 PVC pipe. Cartridges were mounted to the inside wall of the aerosol chamber. Air flow though the cartridges was maintained by diaphragm pumps. Dichotomous TRIG samples were collected for ten minutes on both sides of the cartridge. The dichotomous sampler for TRIG aerosol and vapor was operated and analyzed as previously described.

A model atmosphere of HDI Biuret (Desmodur N-100) and HDI in DMSO, and a representative two-component polyurethane paint based on HDI, Dupont Imron-clear coat, were generated with a DeVilbiss (Sommerset, PA) model 40 nebulizer. The model atmosphere was generated by metering a solution of 5% by weight Desmodur N100 and 1% by volume HDI in DMSO into the nebulizer with a KD Scientific syringe pump, model 200. The syringe pump was operated at a flow of 300 µL per minute. A polypropylene 30-mL Burdick and Jackson syringe containing the appropriate solution was placed in the syringe pump and connected to a 20 gauge needle with a transfer line. The needle was inserted through the vent hole plug of the nebulizer and delivered the solution just below the nebulizer siphon. This configuration provided continuous replacement of nebulized solution and allowed more uniform atmosphere generation. The nebulizer airflow rate was 22 L/min of dried and filtered house air.

Temperature and humidity were monitored over the duration of testing. Temperatures ranged from 21.1 to 25.6° with an average of 22.2° C and relative humidities ranged from 28 to 96% with an average of 46% during the collection of samples. This range reflects those that would be seen in the workplace.

Results

Paired total and respirable particulate samples were collected in the breathing zone of 186 painters in paint shops and painting hangars at five Air Force bases. Using the composition of the starting materials the following formulas were used to estimate maximum TRIG exposure levels.

(1) $\% \ Isocyanate = \dfrac{(w_a)(S_a)(\rho_a)}{[(w_p)(S_p)(\rho_a) + (w_a)(S_a)(\rho_a)]}$

(2) $\% \ Trig = (\% \ Isocyanate)(\% \ NCO \ in \ isocyanate)$

where,
S_a = % Solids by weight of the activator
ρ_a = Density of the activator
w_a = Weighting factor for number of parts activator
S_p = % Solids by weight of the polyol component
ρ_p = Density of the polyol component
w_p = Weighting factor for number of parts polyol
%NCO = (# of Isocyanate groups)(42) / (MW of the isocyanate)

These formulas are based on the following assumptions: 1) The non-solids component of the polyol is completely volatilized 2) The isocyanate is the only solids component of the activator 3) The paint is mixed in the proportions indicated by the instructions.

Table 1-*Estimated Maximum TRIG Levels*

Site	N	Total Aerosol mg/M^3 (geometric mean, σ_g)	Respirable Aerosol mg/M^3 (geometric mean, σ_g)
1	34	1.3, 3.2	0.23, 5.7
2	44	1.2, 2.9	0.12, 2.4
3	43	0.79, 2.3	0.069, 4.4
4	38	0.59, 2.7	0.051, 6.5
5	28	0.59, 2.1	0.094, 6.9

The levels of total aerosol found at each base in paint booths and hangers were compared by Wilcoxon sign rank test and found to be not significantly different (range p>0.13-0.39).

Estimated maximum levels of TRIG for individual sites ranged from 1.3 to 0.59 mg/M^3 for the total aerosol and 0.23 to 0.069 mg/M^3 for the respirable fraction (Table 1). Overall levels were 0.87 mg/M^3 (geometric mean) in the total aerosol and 0.12 mg/M^3 in the respirable fraction with σ_g (geometric standard deviation) of 2.7and 3.3 respectively. The geometric mean of the total TRIG aerosol level was 44 times the recommended HSE TWA for TRIG

Table 2-*Results of Dichotomous Sampling for Aerosols and Vapor of HDI/TRIG during Spray Application of Polyurethane Paint*

Air Sample Volume	Vapor Phase Concentration (μg/M^3)		Aerosol Phase Concentration (μg/M^3)		Activity
(Liters)	HDI	$^+$TRIG	HDI	$^+$TRIG	
20	ND	ND	ND	ND	mixing
20	ND	ND	ND	ND	mixing
150	17	ND	3	551	painting
150	14	ND	5	461	painting
150	7	ND	ND	199	painting
150	10	ND	ND	343	painting
68	2	ND	ND	ND	cleanup/drying
68	5	ND	ND	ND	cleanup/drying
37	ND	ND	ND	ND	cleanup/drying
37	ND	ND	ND	ND	cleanup/drying

$^+$ TRIG: total reactive isocyanate group, reported as equivalent mass of isocyanate (e.g., there are 0.25 μg TRIG per μg HDI). Includes HDI-biuret, other HDI-oligomers, and polyurethane pre-polymers with free isocyanate. Does not include HDI monomer.
ND: not detected (LOD is approximately 0.1 μg HDI / TRIG per sample)

The dichotomous sampler was used to measure vapor and condensed phase TRIG in a paint spray booth. Samples were collected during the mixing of the paint, during the application of a polyurethane paint and during cleanup and drying. The paint spray operations utilized a two part paint based on HDI. Measured levels of TRIG during the spraying operation averaged 391 $\pm$ 154 μg/m^3 (Table 2). This is ~20 times the HSE's recommended TWA for TRIG. Concentrations of HDI averaged only 14 $\pm$ 6.5 μg/m^3,

40% of the American Conference of Governmental Industrial Hygienists (ACGIH) Threshold Limit Value (TLV) of 35 µg/m^3. HDI-biuret was the largest component of TRIG found in these samples and was completely in the condensed aerosol phase. The majority of the HDI was measured in the vapor phase, but significant (15 - 26%) amounts were measured in the aerosol fraction of the paint overspray. After spraying was finished, small amounts of HDI were measured from offgassing of the newly painted surfaces. However, in this case all of the HDI was present in the vapor phase.

Breakthrough of TRIG was examined in a series of APR cartridges. Tests were conducted with a HDI-based two component paint aerosol with median particle size of 1.7 µm and GSD of 2.1 and a model atmosphere, consisting of 1% HDI and 5% Desmodur N100 in dimethylsulfoxide with median particle size of 1.1 µm and GSD of 1.5. Concentrations of TRIG in the test chamber averaged 1318 µg/M^3 and 717 µg/M^3 for the paint and model atmospheres respectively (Table 3).

Table 3- *Chamber Concentrations of TRIG Aerosol*

	Desmodur N100 Test Atmosphere			Paint Test Atmosphere		
	% HDI Vapor	HDI µg/M^3	TRIG µg/M^3	% HDI Vapor	HDI µg/M^3	TRIG µg/M^3
Mean ± σ	82 ± 7	188 ± 91	723 ± 322	ND	ND	1330 ± 344
Range	63-89	120-368	422-1482	ND	ND	493-1732

ND: LOD HDI 0.8 µg/M^3

All the polymeric TRIG was found in the aerosol state. No HDI monomer was detected in the paint atmosphere. In the model atmosphere HDI monomer was present in both vapor and aerosol states. From the dichotomous samplers, it was determined that 82 ± 7 % of the HDI was in the vapor state. This compares well with that seen in the field sampling in the paint booth which showed 78.3 ± 8.6 % of HDI to be in the vapor state during spray painting.

Percent penetration of a particular analyte was determined by comparing its backside cartridge concentration to its chamber concentration. This comparison was done by sample fraction. That is, penetration was evaluated for the cyclone, denuder and back-up filter separately. This would represent penetration by the non-respirable aerosol, vapor phase and respirable aerosol fractions respectively.

$$\%P = {C_b}\big/{C_c} \times 100$$

where:

%P = percent penetration,

C_b = Concentration on the backside of the cartridge, and

C_c = Concentration in the chamber.

Test runs with no cartridge in line show that there was no significant loss of test atmosphere in the system. The percent penetration results for the no cartridge condition had an overall mean and standard deviation of 99.9 ± 2.5 % for TRIG aerosol and 100.2 ± 2.3 % for HDI. No size related bias was observed. Only the backup filter representing the respirable fraction of the aerosol had a level of TRIG greater than the limit of detection for tests run with a cartridge in-line (LOD =3.2 $\mu g/M^3$).

Table 4- *Percentage Penetration of Respirable Fraction of TRIG Aerosol Through APR Cartridge Configurations*

	Desmodur N100 Test Atmosphere	Paint Test Atmosphere	Overall
	(n=6)	(n=6)	n=(12)
	Mean ± σ	Mean ± σ	Mean ± σ
No Cartridge	100.3 ± 4.6	100.3 ± 4.2	100.3 ± 4.4
Organic Vapor Cartridge	72.7 ± 6.0	67.2 ± 3.9	70.0 ± 5.6
Organic Vapor Cartridge with Paint Prefilter	13.5 ± 3.6	13.5 ± 0.6	13.5 ± 2.5
Organic Vapor Cartridge with HEPA Filter	2.7 ± 1.0	2.0 ± 0.5	2.4 ± 0.6

ANOVA Test Results:

Atmosphere p= 0.103

Cartridge p< 0.0001

An analysis of variance of the penetration of respirable TRIG aerosol (Table 4) showed no significant difference in the penetration of the respirable fraction of TRIG between either atmosphere type (p = 0.103). Nor was there a significant interaction between atmosphere and cartridge types ($p = 0.145$).   Respirable TRIG penetration of the cartridges was found to be different from the no cartridge condition and from each other ($p < 0.0001$) by Student-Newman-Keuls test. While the relative percent penetrations across cartridge types were as expected, the magnitudes of the percent penetration were higher than expected. The organic vapor cartridge allowed the penetration of 70% of the respirable TRIG aerosol. The same type of cartridge with a paint prefilter allowed only 13.5 % penetration of the same size fraction. The HEPA / organic vapor cartridge combination provided the best protection, allowing 2.4% of the respirable TRIG aerosol to penetrate. This trend can be seen graphically (Figure 1).

The solution which was used to generate the Desmodur aerosol atmosphere was spiked with 1% HDI monomer. This was done to generate an atmospheric level of HDI monomer of 100 ppb.   For test runs with a cartridge in line, the backside of the cartridge

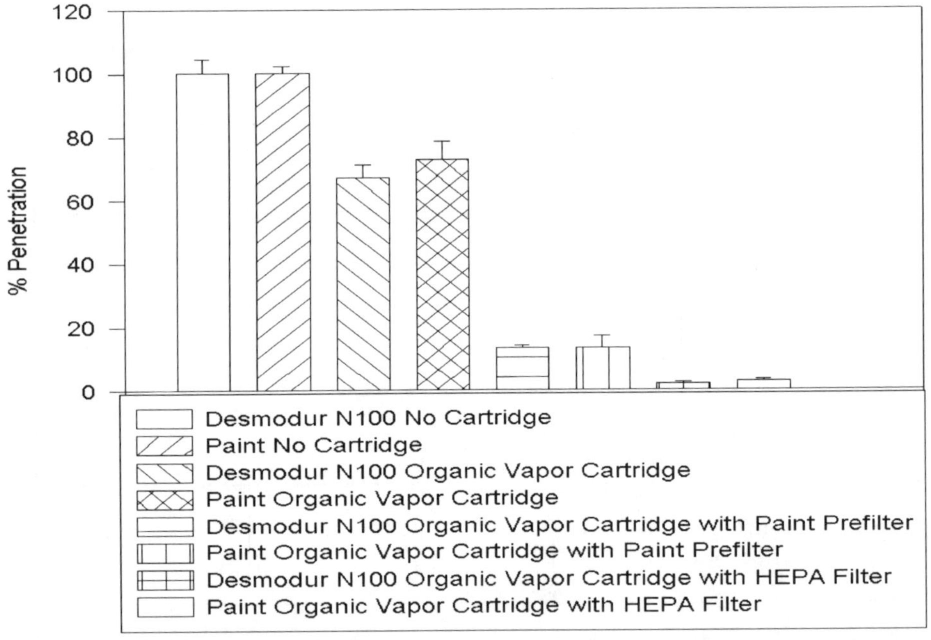

Figure 1 - *Percentage Penetration of Respirable Fraction of TRIG Aerosol Through APR Cartridge Configurations*

showed HDI monomer greater than the LOD only on the backup filter of the dichotomous sampler (Table 5). This would indicate that only aerosol bound HDI monomer penetrated the cartridges. The organic vapor cartridge allowed the penetration of 49.2 % of the aerosol bound HDI monomer. The same type of cartridge with a paint prefilter allowed 21.4 % penetration. The HEPA / organic vapor cartridge combination again provided the best protection, allowing 4.7% of the aerosol to penetrate.

Student-Newman-Kuels T-test showed that each of the cartridges was significantly different from every other cartridge (p < 0.05). The particle size distribution, as determined by Andersen impactor, was significantly smaller by paired T-test (p = 0.03) for the aerosol-bound HDI, MMAD = 0.75 μm, than for the TRIG, MMAD = 1.1 μm. This may account for the apparent increase in penetration of aerosol-bound HDI over TRIG aerosol seen in the paint prefilter and HEPA cartridge configurations.

Table 5- Percentage Penetration of Respirable Fraction of Aerosol-Bound HDI Monomer Through APR Cartridge Configurations

	Desmodur N100 Test Atmosphere	Paint Test Atmosphere
	(n=6)	(n=6)
	Mean ± σ	Mean ± σ
No Cartridge	99.8 ± 3.4	ND
Organic Vapor Cartridge	49.2 ± 10.1	ND
Organic Vapor Cartridge with Paint Prefilter	21.4 ± 5.6	ND
Organic Vapor Cartridge with HEPA Filter	4.7 ± 2.5	ND

Conclusion

Workplace sampling of spray painting operations showed levels of TRIG that exceeded current recommended guidelines. These levels of TRIG indicate the need for engineering controls or protective equipment to prevent overexposure in the workplace. The hangars and a majority of the paint shops utilized either pressure demand respirators or supplied air hoods. This level of protection should be adequate to protect workers for the levels of TRIG exposure estimated from the data. However some of areas studied used half or full face air purifying respirators for protection. The effectiveness of air purifying respirator cartridges in removing TRIG from paint overspray is debatable. Testing was conducted with two aerosol atmospheres: one being a model with the primary TRIG components, HDI monomer and HDI biuret; and the other, an actual polyurethane paint. The chosen atmospheres were designed to represent the worst case scenario for testing the cartridges.   While the relative rates of penetration across cartridge types were as expected, the magnitudes of the penetration rates were higher than expected. The dichotomous sampler data showed that on average, 70% of the respirable TRIG aerosol penetrated the organic vapor cartridge. This lack of protection would raise concerns of over-exposure to workers who used organic vapor cartridges for personal protective equipment in an environment that contained aerosols. The organic vapor cartridge with paint prefilter, with a penetration of 13.5%, significantly improved the collection of respirable particles, but still fell short of the 95% collection efficiency expected of a certified paint / mist filter. The same is true of the organic vapor cartridge with HEPA filter. While 2.4% penetration would be in the range expected of the organic vapor cartridge with paint prefilter, it is less than the 99.97% collection efficiency required for a filter to earn the "High Efficiency" label.

HDI was found to be in the aerosol phase at levels significantly lower than would be expected based on its saturated vapor pressure. This HDI bound aerosol was seen to penetrate the cartrdiges in the same manner as the TRIG aeorsol. The observed penetration of HDI *aerosol* is especially significant in that no HDI *vapor* was seen to penetrate any of the cartridges.

Cartridge testing was conducted prior to the promulgation of the current OSHA respiratory protection standard. This standard carries the new designations of N (nonpresistant), R (resistant) and P (proof) for filters indicating their effectiveness against oil containing aerosols. Determining the efficiency of these different APR cartridge filter combinations and APR cartridges from different manufacturers in removing TRIG would further enhance the accurate selection of respiratory protective equipment for protection against these materials.

Overall, this study suggests that negative pressure air-purifying respirators should not be used for protection against isocyanate containing aerosols. The low levels at which significant health effects can occur, and the inability of any of the cartridge configurations to effectively remove aerosol from the atmosphere, suggest that a high level of risk of over-exposure exists in this practice.

Acknowledgment

This work was supported by grants from the National Institute for Occupational Safety and Health (5R01 OH02664-02), and the Defense Nuclear Agency through the Tulane / Xavier Center for Bioenvironmental Research.

References

[1] Durand, K. T. and Egilman D. S.,"The DuPont Imron Studies: An Example of Possible Misrepresentation of Data in the Industrial Hygiene Literature." *American Industrial Hygiene Association Journal*, 1995, 56 pp.817-825.

[2] Krivanek, N. D, "Response to 'The DuPont Imron Studies: An Example of Possible Misrepresentation of Data in the Industrial Hygiene Literature.'" *American Industrial Hygiene Association Journal*, 1995,56 pp.826-829.

[3] Dhamarajan, V., Lingg R., Hackathron D., "Evaluation of Air-Purifying respirators for Protection Against Toluene Diisocyanate Vapors" *American Industrial Hygiene Association Journal*, 1986, 47 pp.393-398.

[4] Rosenburg, C. and Tuomi T., "Airborne Isocyanates in Polyurethane Spray Painting: Determination and Respirator Efficiency. " *American Industrial Hygiene Association Journal*, 1984, 45 pp.117-121.

[5] Lesage, J., Goyer, N., Desjardins, F., Vincent, J. Y., and Perrault, G., "Worker's Exposure To Isocyanates," *American Industrial Hygiene Association Journal.* 1992, 53 pp.146-153.

[6] Vasta, J. F, "Respirator Cartridge Evaluation for Isocyanate Containing Imron and Centari Enamels." *American Industrial Hygiene Association Journal*, 1985, 46 pp.39-44.

[7] Breslin, P., Occupational Safety and Health Administration, . personal communication with Air Purification Lab, U.S. Divers Company, Santa Ana, CA, May 6, 1982.

[8] Carey,L., Directorate of Field Operations, U.S. Department of Labor, Occupational Safety and Health Administration, Washington D.C. personal communication with W.F. Moon, HSC Corporation, Buchanan, MI, February 20,1987.

[9] Wolfe C., U.S. Department of Labor, Occupational Safety and Health Administration, personal communication with Larry Fack, U.S. Department of Labor, Occupational Safety and Health Administration, Jacksonville, FL, February 15, 1991.

[10] Miles J. B., Jr., Directorate of Field Operations, U.S. Department of Labor, Occupational Safety and Health Administration, Washington D.C., personal communication with Robb Menzies, ACE Systems, Ltd. Lafayette, CO, June 13, 1996.

[11] Weyel D., Ridney B., Alarie Y. "Sensory Irritation. Pulmonary Irritation an Acute Lethality of Polymeric Isocyanate and Sensory Irritation of 2,6 Toluene Diisocyanate" *Toxicology and Applied Pharmacology,* 1982, 644 pp.23-430.

[12] Janko, M., McCarthy K., Fajer M. and van Raalte J., "Occupational Exposure to 1,6-Hexamethylene Diisocyanate-Based Polyisocyanates in the State of Oregon, 1980-1990." *American Industrial Hygiene Association Journal,* 1982, 53 pp.331-338.

[13] Cockcroft, D. W., and Mink J. T., "Isocyanate-induced Asthma in an Automobile Spray Painter," *Canadian Medical Association Journal,* 1979, 121 pp.602-604.

[14] Belin L, Hjortsberg U, Wass U., "Life Threatening Pulmonary Reaction from Car Paint Containing Prepolymerized Isocyanate," *Scandinavian Journal of Work, Environment and Health,* 1981, 7 pp.310-311.

[15] Seguin, P., Allard A., Vartier A.and Malo J., "Prevalence of Occupational Asthma in Spray Painters Exposed to Several Types of Isocyanates, Including Polymethylene Polyphenylisocyanate." *Journal of Occupational Medicine,* 1987, 29(4) pp.340-344.

[16] Nielsen J, Sango C, Winroth G, Hallberg T, Skerfving S,. "Systemic Reactions Associated with Polyisocyanate Exposure," *Scandinavian Journal of Work, Environment and Health,* 1985, 11 pp.51-54.

[17] Alexandersson R., Plato N., Kolmodin-Hedman B. and Hedenstierna G., "Exposure, Lung Function, and Symptoms in Car Painters Exposed to Hexamethylendiisocyanate and Biuret Modified Hexamethylene Diisocyanate," *Archives of Environmental Health* 1987, 42 pp.367-373.

[18] Tornling G., Alexandersson R., Hedenstiera G. and Plato N., " Decreased Lung Function and Exposure to Diisocyanates (HDI and HDI-BT) in Car Repair Painters: Observations on Re-examination 6 Years After Initial Study." *American Journal of Industrial Medicine,* 1990, 17 pp.299-310.

[19] Rando, R. J., Poovey, H. G., "Development And Application Of A Dichotomous Vapor/Aerosol Sampler For HDI-Derived Total Reactive Isocyanate Group," *American Industrial Hygiene Association Journal,* 1999, 60 pp.737-746.

[20] Silverman, L., Lee G., Plotkin T., Sawyers L. and Yancey A, "Air Flow Measurements on Human Subjects with and without Respiratory Resistance at Several Work Rates" *Industrial Hygiene and Occupational Medicine,* 1951, 3 pp.461-478.

Stefanie M. Corbitt[1] E.A. Heger[2] David G. Sarvadi[3]

Use of Air-Purifying Respirators for Substances with Limited or Poor Warning Properties

---

Reference: Corbitt, S. M., Heger, E. A., and Sarvadi, D. G., **"Use of Air-Purifying Respirators for Substances with Limited or Poor Warning Properties,"** *Isocyanates: Sampling, Analysis, and Health Effects, ASTM STP 1408,* J. Lesage, I. D. DeGraff, and R. S. Danchik, Eds., American Society for Testing and Materials, West Conshohocken, PA, 2002.

Abstract: In 1998, the Occupational Safety and Health Administration (OSHA) updated its general industry respiratory protection standard, 29 C.F.R. § 1910.134. The use of air-purifying respirators (APR) was affected by a significant policy change that requires employers to provide respirators equipped with a NIOSH certified end-of-service-life indicator (ESLI) for the expected contaminant, or to implement a change schedule for canisters and cartridges based on objective data showing that the cartridges are effective in preventing exposure to the contaminant, and have an adequate service life.

However, questions continue to be raised about the permissibility of using APR in certain industrial applications where workers may be exposed above allowable limits to substances with poor warning properties. This paper outlines some of the important considerations such as: what data are necessary to demonstrate that the respirator cartridge/filter is quantitatively effective at removing the contaminant of interest, and what data are needed to demonstrate that employee exposures to a contaminant are within the range that the respirator can effectively remove it from the inhaled air stream. These considerations must be taken into account to assure that APR are properly selected and used to provide protection against substances with poor warning properties. Methylenediphenyl diisocyanate (MDI) and polymeric products made from MDI will be used as an example in this discussion.

Keywords: air-purifying respirators, change out schedule, OSHA, NIOSH, MDI, poor warning properties, chemical exposure, hazardous chemical exposure, and isocyanates, ESLI odor threshold, respiratory protection.

---

[1] OSHA Regulatory Specialist, Keller & Heckman LLP, 1001 G Street, NW, Suite 500W, Washington, DC, 20001.

[2] Pesticide Registration Manager, Keller & Heckman LLP, 1001 G Street, NW, Suite 500W, Washington, DC, 20001.

[3] Attorney and Certified Industrial Hygienist, Keller & Heckman LLP, 1001 G Street, NW, Suite 500W, Washington, DC, 20001.

Introduction

Historically, both the National Institute for Occupational Safety and Health (NIOSH) and the Occupational Safety and Health Administration (OSHA)[1] adopted standard industry practice by prohibiting the use against gases and vapors of air-purifying respirators (APR) that have inadequate warning properties — principally where the odor threshold is above the applicable exposure limit. Generally, APR could only be used in situations where (1) an adequate oxygen supply (greater than 19.5%) is available; (2) the atmosphere is not Immediately Dangerous to Life and Health (IDLH); and (3) for vapors and gases, the chemical has suitable warning properties to allow the respirator user to detect failure of the filtration or adsorption cartridge. Diisocyanates are an example of a class of chemicals that made it impossible for APR to be used to protect against overexposure, because the odor thresholds are above the applicable exposure limits.

The rationale for the prohibition was simple. Respirators designed for controlling exposures to airborne vapors and gases by filtration or chemical removal of contaminants generally did not incorporate a means of determining when the capacity of the cartridge had been exceeded. The principal method of detecting leakage of the chemical through the cartridge, odor, is dependent on two factors: the ability of the wearer to detect the contaminant, and the odor threshold being below the allowable exposure limit. For example, the odor thresholds for diisocyanates are above the respective PELs and TLVs of 0.02 ppm and 0.005 ppm. Accordingly, OSHA issued several statements over the last 20 years to the effect that APR with chemical cartridges were not "approved" for use against diisocyanates, and, therefore, APR could not be used where respiratory protection was needed to control exposures above the PEL or TLV[4].

---

[4] Respiratory Protection Program Manual OSHA Directives - CPL 2-2.54, 02/10/1992. OSHA Standards Interpretation and Compliance Letters, e.g., The use of negative-pressure air-purifying respirators for protection against paint spray containing isocyanates. 01/25/1985; Respirator Concern, 06/13/1996, and Respirator use in spray operations involving paints containing isocyanates, 07/11/1994. In spite of these considerations, it has been shown that where diisocyanates were present in conjunction with organic solvents, the solvents typically had shorter breakthrough times than the diisocyanates, and with lower odor thresholds, could be used to indicate when cartridges should be changed. Nevertheless, OSHA balked at agreeing that the APR could be used to protect against diisocyanate exposure. See, The use of negative-pressure air-purifying respirators for protection against paint spray containing isocyanates 01/25/1985.

Requirements of the Revised OSHA Respiratory Protection Standard

On January 8, 1998, OSHA published a final rule on Respiratory Protection, replacing the regulations set forth at 29 C.F.R. § 1910.134 [2]. The standard applies to all respirator use in general industry, shipyards, marine terminals, longshoring, and construction workplaces. Under the new rules, employers had until October 5, 1998, to comply with the revised standard. This standard applies when (1) employees are required to wear respirators to protect themselves from exposure to air contaminants above a specific exposure limit, (2) if the employer requires respirators to be worn, or (3) if respirators are otherwise necessary to protect employee health. Additionally, limited requirements apply when employees, for personal, comfort, or other reasons, voluntarily choose to wear certain kinds of APR. The standard affirms OSHA's long-standing policy that personal protective equipment — in this instance, respirators — are to be the last line of defense when engineering and work practice controls are inadequate to reduce employee exposure, or during the development and installation of other controls.

Among other requirements, the standard mandates that employers:

- Develop a written program;
- Assign a program administrator;
- Prepare work site-specific procedures;
- Select respirators on the basis of the hazard present and the protection required;
- Train employees in the use and limitations of respirators;
- Fit test employees;
- Provide medical evaluation; and,
- Provide for respirator cleaning, maintenance, and repair.

A major change in the standard is the provision governing when APR may be used. The new standard permits the use of APR without limit, *if* the employer has objective data (1) that APR provide adequate protection, and (2) on the service life of the cartridges, upon which a cartridge change out schedule may be based. Generally, half-mask APR are assigned a protection factor of 10 or less, while full-face APR may be assigned a PF of 50, and powered air purifying respirators (PAPR) may have a 25-100 PF. (*American National Standard for Respiratory Protection*. ANSI, Z88.2-1992. New York, NY. There is controversy and uncertainty over the correct PF to assign APR. The decision depends on how much leakage occurs, not on the efficiency of the filtration devices in most cases. For particulate filters, the efficiencies can be in excess of 1000 or more, while field studies suggest that overall PF can be as low as 2-5. Whatever the case, the data presented here show that efficiency factors not related to fit are more than adequate to provide a reasonable degree of protection against diisocyanates. See, OSHA Standard Discussion, supra. p 9-11.) Accordingly, such devices usually will be acceptable, assuming adequate supporting data, in workplaces where airborne levels are up to ten to one hundred times the permissible exposure limit or the ACGIH TLV.

The standard provides what we consider exceptionally clear and unambiguous guidance on what employers are supposed to do in implementing a program using APR to protect against gas and vapor exposure. The key language in 29 C.F.R. § 1910.134(d)(3)(iii) states:

> "For protection against gases and vapors, the employer shall implement . . . a change schedule for canisters and cartridges that is based on objective information or data that will ensure that canisters and cartridges are changed before the end of their service life. The employer shall describe in the respirator program the information and data relied upon and the basis for the canister and cartridge change schedule and the basis for reliance on the data"*[3]*.

OSHA further explained what it expected in regard to development of change schedules in the following language from the *Federal Register*:

> ". . . [T]he requirement in the final rule would not require the employer to search for and analyze breakthrough test data, but instead permits the employer to obtain information from other sources who have the expertise and knowledge to be able to assist the employer to develop change schedules. OSHA has revised the final rule from the proposal in this manner to recognize that there may be instances in which specific breakthrough test data are not available for a particular contaminant, but manufacturers and suppliers may nevertheless still be able to provide guidance to an employer to develop an adequate change schedule. If the employer is unable to obtain such data, information, or recommendations to support the use of air-purifying respirators against the gases or vapors encountered in the employer's workplace, the final rule requires the employer to rely on atmosphere-supplied respirators because the employer can have no assurance that air-purifying respirators will provide adequate protection"*[3]*.

And later in the Preamble, OSHA further states:

> "If breakthrough data are not available, the employer may seek other information on which to base a reliable cartridge/canister change schedule. OSHA believes that the most readily available alternative is for employers to rely on recommendations of their respirator and/or chemical suppliers. To be reliable, such recommendations should consider *workplace-specific* factors that are likely to affect cartridge/canister service life, such as concentrations of contaminants in the workplace air, patterns of respirator use (i.e., whether use is intermittent or continuous throughout the shift), and environmental factors including temperature and humidity. [Emphasis added]"*[3]*.

Due to differences in respirators, individuals, and site factors, employers generally must perform a site-specific evaluation to estimate the service life of cartridges. However, that site-specific evaluation can be based, in part, on data from other sources. OSHA states that:

> "Exposures must be characterized, through methods that may include actual measurements of exposure at a worksite, *exposure data from industry or suppliers*, and calculations of concentration based on amount used (mathematical models). Data from industry-wide surveys by trade associations may be used as long as they *closely resemble* the processes and work conditions as described in the survey. The standard does not specify how an employer is to make a reasonable estimate, nor does it require the employer to measure employee exposure. Even with actual measurements of exposure, some estimation is still

involved, since monitoring only determines the exposure on a particular day for a specific employee [emphasis added]"[3].

Thus, it is clear that OSHA expects associations and other industry groups working together will develop general guidelines and data on anticipated exposures, suitable respirators and cartridge change schedules for specific chemicals. Regardless of its source, the data must support the conclusion that (1) the device provides adequate protection, subject to the general limitations on APR with regard to fit and face piece seal leakage, and (2) the cartridge or filter removes the intended contaminant, providing adequate protection for a suitable period of time that is known and predictable. In general, we would expect OSHA to interpret the term "adequate protection" to mean that taking into account the potential exposure and the PF of the respirator, use of the APR lowers the concentration of the contaminant in the inhaled air stream to below the applicable PEL or TLV.

Policy Change at NIOSH

In 1999, NIOSH reexamined its policies on respirator usage to address this and several other issues that were thrown into question by OSHA's final standard. On August 4, 1999, the Respirator Use Policy Workgroup issued a policy statement to conform NIOSH's policies with OSHA's new standard in five areas [4]. One of these was the question of reliance on warning properties, and the use and development of change schedules for chemical cartridges. NIOSH decided to "update its policy to be consistent with OSHA by recognizing the use of change schedules and by recommending *against* reliance on warning properties [emphasis added]".

Significantly, NIOSH stated that the uncertainties of change schedules are less significant than continued reliance on warning properties. NIOSH recounted some of the problems with warning properties: wide variation in odor thresholds in the general population; shift in odor threshold due to extended low exposures; shifts due to personal factors (colds, allergies, etc.); failure to recognize odor due to distractions; and inaccuracies in determining employee sensitivity to odor. NIOSH noted that the efficacy of change schedules has not been documented, but recognized that improved methods of developing change schedules would develop over time. Also, NIOSH called for additional research "to develop and validate clear and practical methods for employers to establish change schedules." Thus, it is clear that prior NIOSH policies against the use of APR with substances having poor warning properties are no longer valid. Implementing this change, NIOSH is revising "Caution H" that is printed on respirator approvals for APR. If APR are to be used in accordance with NIOSH policy, the new language will require that users "follow established cartridge and canister change schedules or observe ESLI to ensure that cartridges and canisters are replaced before breakthrough occurs."

A Case Study Using Methylenediphenyl Diisocyanate (MDI)

MDI is used in manufacturing a variety of polyurethane products. It is also reacted with cellulosics, rubbers, and phenolics to produce products such as oriented strand board, athletic surfaces, and foundry cores and molds [5].

For manufacturers to comply with OSHA's new procedure, they must demonstrate that APR are effective at removing the contaminant quantitatively from the inhaled air stream for a suitable period of time. In the case of diisocyanates, this work has already been completed. On OSHA's web site are data showing that organic vapor cartridges combined with particulate filters provide more than adequate protection against exposures to aerosols of MDI and its oligomers. The paper by Spence et al [6], shows beyond doubt that such devices remove MDI particulate and vapor from the inhaled air stream, when challenged with concentrations far exceeding current exposure limits. The data indicate that organic vapor cartridges with dust/mist (DM) or high efficiency particulate (HEPA) filters effectively removed greater than 99% of MDI aerosol and vapor in all test atmospheres. Further, breakthrough times for spray-generated MDI aerosols using the above noted particulate filters, in series with the organic vapor cartridge, occurred at greater than 24 hours with a detection limit of approximately 1 ppb (10 μg/m^3). The effective service life of a properly selected respirator combination, according to the data from the study, is more than 24 hours.

The data support the conclusion that chemical cartridges containing activated charcoal combined with particulate filters remove diisocyanates from the inhaled air stream with breakthrough times in excess of 24 hours, when the inhaled air stream contains concentrations no higher than 10 000 ppb (10 ppm). This is equivalent to 500 times the OSHA PEL, or 2000 times the ACGIH TLV for MDI. Generally accepted industry guidance indicates that APR should not be used in situations where exposure to a contaminant exceeds a level equal to the PF for the type of respirator; e.g., ten times the TLV (or PEL for legal compliance) for a half mask respirator. Accordingly, these data support the conclusion that the combination APR described above is quantitatively efficient against MDI and that the service life is sufficiently long to establish a cartridge/filter change schedule of eight hours (or possibly more). However, to prevent abuse and potential overuse of the cartridge, we suggest limiting use to a maximum service life of 8 hours. Thus, under OSHA's standard, if an employer shows that exposures to airborne levels of MDI in its operations are less than 500 times the PEL, or below 2500 ppb (5.0 * 500) time-weighted-average (TWA) or 10 000 ppb ceiling or Short Term Exposure Limit (STEL), these data allow the use of a combination half-mask APR to protect against inhalation of airborne MDI. If an employer has data showing that its employees are exposed to levels below those used as challenge concentrations in this study up to the maximum levels cited above, the employer may rely on the data in the Spence et al [7] paper to comply with this provision of the standard.

"Polymeric MDI" or crude MDI is used in many industrial applications. "Polymeric MDI" is a mixture of 4,4' MDI, 2,4' MDI, and a number of polymerized diisocyanates where the repeating structural unit is a benzyl diisocyanate group. The polymeric MDI usually contains 50% 4,4' MDI monomer, and varying amounts of MDI-polymers with n = 1 to about 10; the amount of polymerization decreases with increasing number of n. The isocyanate (-NCO) functional group in the polymers can be in the -ortho, -meta or -para positions [7].

Both polymeric MDI (PMDI) and MDI have very low vapor pressures. Thus, there is limited potential for exposure to airborne vapor at normal ambient temperatures [9]. For both products, the vapor pressure is such that, at ambient temperature and pressure, the maximum theoretical concentration in air for pure MDI is in the range of 7-64 ppb, and is correspondingly lower for complex mixtures and for PMDI [8] [5]. Actual measurements in operations using PMDI confirm that airborne concentrations are low. Hence, on a theoretical basis alone, an APR equipped with a particulate filter and appropriate organic vapor cartridge and having a protection factor of 10 should be adequate to protect against exposure to airborne MDI or related polymeric materials under normal conditions of use. These measurements also show that, under certain conditions, high exposures can be found. The Alliance for the Polyurethanes Industry is supporting additional work to prepare this information for publication in the near future.

For many years, publications of the Alliance for the Polyurethanes Industry only recommended the use of air-supplied respirators in polyurethane applications, especially in applications where particulate aerosols are generated [9]. For products containing low-molecular-weight diisocyanates such as MDI, such recommendations were reasonable. This recommendation can now be modified.

Two considerations must be addressed in deciding whether to rescind the recommendation for air-supplied respirators. First, is exposure to isocyanate-containing vapor likely? Second, if so, are air-purifying respirators adequate to protect against any such vapor exposure? We take each of these in turn.

Vapor exposures are unlikely to be significant. As noted above, theoretical limits on vapor exposure mean the only possible exposures at ambient temperatures are very low. In most spray applications, for example, although some vapor might be present, the principal potential exposure is to particulate aerosol that may have reactive isocyanate groups on the molecules. Although vapor exposures theoretically can occur where the MDI-containing product is heated significantly above ambient temperatures, for PMDI products, significant vapor exposure is unlikely, assuming the law of potential pressures applies, because the vapor pressure of MDI is so low, even with a significant fraction of MDI in the product.

Second, the data cited above show that the particulate/vapor cartridge removes all isocyanate from the inhaled air stream, and for a sufficient period of time to allow change schedules to be used effectively. Thus, it is reasonable to conclude that (1) respiratory protection against inhalation of diisocyanate *vapor* is not necessary in most applications using PMDI and (2) except in unusual situations (heating of the resin), *particulate* respirators will provide adequate protection against inhalation of isocyanate in contaminated air. Thus, the manufacturers of MDI-containing products now can recommend that appropriate respirators consisting of organic vapor cartridges and high

---

[5] The vapor pressure of a PMDI/MDI mixture can be estimated by applying adjustment factors to the vapor pressure of MDI, based on the percentage of MDI in the mixture.

efficiency filters be used where direct exposure to potential airborne concentrations of diisocyanates, in whatever form, can occur.

However, there is no longer a theoretical basis for prohibiting the use of APR having an adequate particulate filter and chemical cartridge capable of capturing organic vapors to protect against exposure to MDI. Where there are other contaminants present, the APR should be equipped with a suitable chemical cartridge to remove those substances, in combination with the particulate filter/OV cartridge, and the cartridge change schedule should be adjusted to account for the efficiency of the combination against the chemical mixture. In the absence of a suitable cartridge/filter combination, APR should not be used.

Environmental and operating variables affect the amount of diisocyanate generated in a particular workplace atmosphere as well as the function and efficiency of respirators. The method and rate of application directly affects the airborne concentrations, as does the amount of water in the air, the amount and kind of ventilation present, and the physical layout of the area in which the product is applied. Spray application increases the potential for diisocyanate exposure due to formation of liquid and solid aerosols (particulates), as does an increase in the ambient temperature and humidity at the time of application *[10]*. As the relative humidity and temperature rise, a larger quantity of water vapor will compete with the diisocyanate for the adsorbent found in the cartridges *[11]*. Generally, in areas with restricted airflow or where open doors or windows create cross-drafts that may increase potential exposure by blowing high concentrations toward the user, airborne levels will be higher. Lastly, there may be other chemicals that interfere with the cartridge's ability to absorb diisocyanate.

Other factors that affect the concentrations to which employees are exposed include:
1. the characteristics of the respirator in use;
2. human factors, including respiration rate (as influenced by work rate), respirator to face seal, cleanliness of the respirator; and
3. use of other personal protective equipment.

These factors *determine the amount of* diisocyanates an employee wearing a respirator actually breathes. For example, if employees are working at high metabolic rates, their respiration rates will increase proportionately. Canisters and cartridges have a limited amount of adsorbent to trap the diisocyanates. Thus, on a theoretical basis alone, an employee breathing twice the usual working rate could consume the cartridge capacity and saturate the cartridge in half the normal time. Additionally, cartridges manufactured by different companies may vary in the amount of MDI and PMDI absorbed.

All of the above factors must be considered when deciding whether to rely on the data on breakthrough times and to estimate potential exposures in any particular workplace. To the extent that the employer can reasonably conclude that its operations are similar to other operations, then data from the similar operations may be used to develop change schedules. If the employer has some, but perhaps not a substantial amount of exposure data, there are no unusual operations, and the data show measurements below 200 ppb, the employer may conclude that the potential exposure will not exceed 195 ppb and that APR having a protection factor of 10 may be used to protect employees against airborne levels of MDI.

Employers may also need to provide air-supplied respirators when employees apply PMDI in spraying applications and when there are extended work periods required in atmospheres that are not IDLH. In the absence of data, employers should assume that air supplied respirators are required. The assigned protection factor for air-supplied respirators is usually 1000 or greater. While provision of an air-supplied respirator also requires compliance with the OSHA respiratory protection standard, there is a substantially larger margin of safety. However, employers must take into account the extra effort and hazards associated with the use of air-supplied systems, and should balance these considerations, along with estimated exposures, in deciding whether APR or air-supplied systems are provided.

Conclusions and Recommendations

The change in OSHA's policy, coupled with the publication of data on the efficacy of APR against methylenediphenyl diisocyanate (MDI)- containing atmospheres, now permits the use of APR in certain circumstances. OSHA has recently confirmed this interpretation in a letter to the authors responding to questions submitted on behalf of the industry trade association, the Alliance for the Polyurethanes Industry (API) *[12]*. The letter reminds users that many significant steps must be taken to assure that respirators are properly used and selected, but confirms that APR can be used to provide protection against substances like diisocyanates where odor thresholds are below acceptable exposure levels. In addition, OSHA indicated that it would be reviewing other documents on its web site and in its files that provide contradictory advice and will be revising those policy statements accordingly *[13]*.

When APR test data are combined with statistically significant field or laboratory sample data, we conclude that such devices can be used with confidence to provide protection against substances with limited or poor warning properties, and afford compliance with the new OSHA respiratory protection standard.

Acknowledgments

The authors wish to thank The Alliance for the Polyurethanes Industry, a business unit of the American Plastics Council, for the sponsorship of this publication.

References

[1] Regulations predating the January 1998 OSHA Revision, 63 *Fed. Reg.* 1152, Jan. 8, 1998.

[2] 63 *Fed. Reg.* 1152, Jan. 8, 1998.

[3] "Questions and Answers on the Respiratory Protection Standard, August 3, 1998 OSHA Memorandum from John B. Miles to All Regional Administrators. " [Online] http://www.osha-slc.gov/SLTC/respiratory_advisor/oshafiles/require.html. (Accessed Sept. 15, 2000).

[4] "NIOSH Respirator Use Policy Statement," URL: http://www.khlaw.com/NIOSH2.pdf, Keller & Heckman LLP website, material provided by NIOSH, 200 Independence Ave., SW, Room 715H, Washington, DC, 4 August 1999.

[5] George Woods: *The ICI Polyurethanes Book.* Chichester: John Wiley & Sons, 1990.

[6] Spence, M.W., T.D. Landry, and D.W. Huff: "Evaluation of the Effectiveness of Air-purifying Respirator Cartridges in Removing MDI Aerosols from Air." URL: http://www.osha-slc.gov/SLTC/isocyanates/mdi/mdi.html, OSHA Website, material provided by Dow Chemical Company, Midland, MI.

[7] Levine, S.P., K.J.D. Hillig, V. Dharmarajan, M.W. Spence, M.D. Baker: Critical Review of Methods of Sampling, Analysis, and Monitoring for TDI and MDI. *American Industrial Hygiene Association Journal* 56(6):581–589 (1995).

[8] *Alliance for the Polyurethanes Industry' Guide to Reporting MDI Emissions under EPCRA.* Appendix A, 2000.

[9] Polyurethane Division/The Society of the Plastics Industry, Inc., MDI-based Polyurethane Foam Systems: Guidelines for Safe Handling and Disposal.*Technical Bulletin AZ119,* November 1993.

[10] Review of the OSHA web page can provide additional information, URL: http://www.osha-slc.gov/SLTC/respiratoryprotection/index.html.

[11] OSHA's "Rule of Thumb" page suggests that humidity above 85% will reduce service life by 50%, URL: http://www.osha-slc.gov/SLTC/respiratoryprotection/index.html

[12] Department of Labor Letter to Mr. David Sarvadi, June 18, 2000, URL:
   http://www.polyurethane.org/project_stewardship/respirators.PDF

$54.00

SBA
14/05